Genomes, Molecular Biology and Drug Discovery

Genomes, Molecular Biology and Drug Discovery

Edited by

M. J. BROWNE

SmithKline Beecham Pharmaceuticals
New Frontiers Science Park
Harlow, Essex

and

P. L. THURLBY

SmithKline Beecham Pharmaceuticals
New Frontiers Science Park
Harlow, Essex

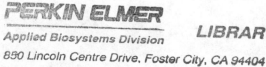

ACADEMIC PRESS

Harcourt Brace & Company, Publishers

London   San Diego   New York
Boston   Sydney   Tokyo   Toronto

ACADEMIC PRESS LIMITED
24–28 Oval Road
LONDON NW1 7DX

United States Edition published by
ACADEMIC PRESS INC.
San Diego, CA 92101

A catalogue record for this book is available from the British Library
ISBN 0-12-137790-3

Typeset by Phoenix Photosetting, Chatham, Kent
Printed in Great Britain by Hartnolls Ltd, Bodmin, Cornwall

Contents

II   INTERPRETING THE CODE

III   FROM GENE TO TARGET

IV   FROM TARGET TO THERAPY

10   Monoclonal Antibodies: Tools for Exploiting Gene Discovery   151
D. P. Bloxham

11   Retroviral Vectors: First-Generation Systems for Gene Therapy   165
D. E. Onions

Appendix: Abstracts of Posters   **179**

Index   **191**

A colour plate section can be found between pages 84 and 85.

Contributors

M. D. Adams   The Institute for Genomic Research, 9712 Medical Center Drive, Rockville, MD 20850, USA

D. P. Bloxham   Chief Executive Officer, Celltech Therapeutics Ltd, 216 Bath Road, Slough, Berks SL1 4EN, UK

J. C. Chabala   President and Chief Scientific Officer, Pharmacopeia, Inc., 101 College Road East, Princeton, NJ 08540, USA

J.-M. Claverie   CNRS-EP91, Information Génétique et Moléculaire, IBSM, 31 Chemin Joseph Aiguier, 13402 Marseille Cedex 20, France

F. Grosveld   MGC Department of Cell Biology and Genetics, Erasmus Universiteit, Rotterdam, The Netherlands

J.-L. Guenet   Institut Pasteur, 25 rue du Dr Roux, 75724 Paris, Cedex 15, France

P. Little   Department of Biochemistry, Imperial College, Imperial College Road, London SW7 2AZ, UK

D. E. Onions   Department of Veterinary Pathology, University of Glasgow, The Veterinary School, Bearsden Road, Bearsden, Glasgow G61 1QH, UK

A. R. Shatzman   SmithKline Beecham Pharmaceuticals, 709 Swedeland Road, King of Prussia, PA 19406-2799, USA

M. J. E. Sternberg   Biomolecular Modelling Laboratory, Imperial Cancer Research Fund, 44 Lincoln's Inn Fields, London WC2A 3PX, UK

P. J. Whiting   Neuroscience Research Centre, Merck Sharp and Dohme Research Laboratories, Terlings Park, Harlow, Essex CM20 2QR, UK

Introduction

Genomes, Molecular Biology and Drug Discovery, Cambridge,
March 1995

In one of the most rapidly moving fields in biological and medical sciences, this
Symposium focuses on how the continuing advances in modern genome research
and molecular biology, combined with new pharmacological and chemical strategies, will help to realize the achievement of practical therapeutic endpoints.

This book is based on the 7th SmithKline Beecham International Symposium, held
at Robinson College, Cambridge in March 1995. These symposia are devoted to
addressing ground-breaking advances in scientific research. However, whilst organizing the symposium we realized that the programme would need to be radically different from its predecessors. In previous years it had been usual and indeed reasonable
to focus on one scientific discipline. With the increasing progress being made by the
'genome projects' we recognized that pharmaceutical research had reached a water-
shed and now was the time to take a broad look at what the various genome projects
would be capable of delivering. However there was a critical difference between this
and other 'genome meetings'—we felt a need to examine how that wealth of information could actually be used to generate new therapeutics: ultimately to deliver
superior and better targeted healthcare to the community. In many ways the conference paralleled the 'real life issues' faced by academic, pharmaceutical and healthcare institutions in truly realizing the benefits from the genome projects.

The challenge to the speakers was not only to deliver first rate science but also to
deliver it in the context of the need to break down barriers between scientific disciplines—this will be required if we are finally to benefit, in a tangible sense, from the
increasing number of genes being identified.

Until recently, genes have been cloned and expressed usually as the result of targeted programmes of research. The new genes were then expressed, biochemistry
and pharmacology evaluated, high throughput mechanism-based screens were
devised and leads identified for optimization by medical chemists—yielding the
many therapeutic agents we are familiar with that are already in the clinic or in
development.

In this, by now traditional, model of pharmaceutical research, gene identification had often been considered rate-limiting. The paradigm has suddenly shifted. As a result of the 'genome projects', we now see new gene sequences being identified on a scale that would have been unimaginable 10 years ago. Pharmaceutical research needs rapidly to come to terms with this dramatically altered situation. For example, we need to be able to use the raw sequence data to predict which genes may be useful and why. Molecular biologists and protein chemists are being confronted with a flood of genes to express and purify; pharmacologists and biochemists are facing greater challenges in assigning functionality to new proteins, either new members of established protein families or sometimes entirely novel proteins. Additionally as there are potentially many, many more proteins to work with, the abundance of opportunities is suddenly beginning to impact on conventional research strategies. The 'high throughput' screening teams need to accommodate an increased number of potential targets, medicinal chemists need to be able to elaborate new pharmacologically active agents on an unprecedented scale, the protein engineer now has a wider range of potential protein therapeutic agents to manipulate and develop via clinical trials. On the horizon, gene therapy, though confronted with technical challenges, seems increasingly to be a logical route to treatment of many diseases, not only the single gene defects but also many common multifactorial diseases with a strong genetic component.

A key feature of this new 'functional continuum' will be the need to establish quickly and unambiguously the *in vivo* functionality of targets deriving from the 'gene first' strategy. Above all, the individual scientific disciplines need to work with far greater integration and a greater sense of identity with the overall process that will take us from a 'string of nucleotides in a database' to radically new therapies.

Though the genome projects offer a greater choice of pharmacological targets, at the same time we are aware that the scientific community has to be responsive to increasing economic pressures, which are driving down research funds, and the increasing demand for measurable improvements in the 'pharmaco-economic outcome' of new treatments. The genome projects are thus providing radically new opportunities, but to make the most of these opportunities our downstream research processes need simultaneously to improve in terms of technology and in better organization to deliver worthwhile results in ever-decreasing time scales.

That 'genome science' has a central part to play in pharmaceutical research can no longer be in any serious doubt: many major pharmaceutical companies have launched large in-house genome efforts and several have announced multi-million dollar research alliances. SmithKline Beecham was the first via its collaboration with Human Genome Sciences: others followed, including Pfizer and Upjohn with Incyte and Merck with Washington University.

The next decade will be a truly exciting period in the evolution of pharmaceutical research. We are confident that we will look back in 10 years with the realization that the changes, initially driven by genome research, have in fact thoroughly revolutionized the way in which novel drugs are identified and developed.

MICHAEL J. BROWNE AND
PETER THURLBY

I

GENOME PROJECTS

1

The Human Genome Project: What We Want and What We Get

PETER LITTLE

*Department of Biochemistry, Imperial College,
London SW7 2AZ, UK*

Abstract

The goal of the genome project is to understand the information content of our DNA: the primary structure of proteins is only a single component of this information and we also need to know the sequence of promoter elements and the sequence context in which genes and promoter elements are embedded. We know from a number of gene systems that locus control regions can be quite distant from the genes they influence: this implies that sequencing the immediate environment of genes is not a sufficient analysis. Evidence is accumulating that DNA sequence along chromosomal sized domains is far from homogeneous since gene clustering, deviation from expected base composition and clustered distribution of repetitive elements are well described. This would appear to point towards dynamics that can only reasonably be addressed by a more detailed description of sequence. Sequence dynamics are likely to be of some importance in considerations of the evolution of the control of gene expression: this again argues that we need to establish the sequence of the whole genome and that we do not have a sufficiently sophisticated understanding of DNA to allow us to select more limited regions for analysis.

There has been much discussion of how complete and accurate DNA sequence analysis must be within the projects described above. There is no one 'sequence' of the genome: base variants occur at a frequency of 1 in 100 bp to 1 in 1000 bp in humans and analysis of human variance, be it mutations associated with disease, with polymorphisms or structural instability, are a key feature of most human molecular genetic analyses. This suggests that absolute accuracy in sequence determination is an irrelevance: what we need is sufficiently accurate information to know what the general properties of a sequence are, i.e. the likely presence of exons, repeats, base composition clustering and so forth. This will lead investigators into the sequence analysis of multiple isolates of the same region, addressing the

GENOMES, MOLECULAR BIOLOGY AND DRUG DISCOVERY
ISBN 0-12-137790-3

problem of variance directly, as well as establishing a truly 'accurate' sequence of the region.

1 The genome project

The human genome project (HGP) has always been thought of progressing as a series of increasingly detailed analyses of the genome which would culminate, ultimately, in the direct determination of complete sequence in perhaps 2005. The long time scale and the very considerable sums of money involved have allowed a number of interim goals to achieve greater prominence than otherwise would have been the case. In this article, I review what we require out of the genome project, what has been achieved so far, what interim goals have been set, how these do or do not meet the scientific aims of the HGP and review how our own work on chromosome 11 is a reasonable exemplar of the immediate problems facing genome workers. I have deliberately focused on the human genome; it is important to recognize that the results of other genome projects, including *Escherichia coli,* yeast, *Caenorhabditis elegans*, mouse and *Drosophila*, are absolutely central to the interpretation and exploitation of human genomic data.

1.1 The goals

The explicit aims of the HGP are rarely defined in discussions of the project: I believe that it is important to do so since a clear definition shows that many activities are either partial solutions to the problems of the project or are intermediate goals. I would define the final goals of the HGP as the identification of the following features of human DNA.

(i) The presence of genes at defined locations in the genome.
(ii) The sequence and structure of the genes, including exon/intron structure and motifs.
(iii) Promoter structure, including sequence classes of promoter and a catalogue of transcription factor binding sites.
(iv) The sequence environment of the gene—GC or AT rich?
(v) The structure of the intergenic DNA—base composition asymmetries, repeat distributions, higher order structures and local repeats.

1.2 The strategies

Strategies leading up to the complete determination of sequence have evolved over the last 5 years: in summary, the approach that has been developed is to generate detailed recombination or radiation hybrid maps of markers (Weissenbach *et al.,* 1992; James *et al.,* 1994; Gyapay *et al.,* 1994). The approach makes major use of polymerase chain reaction (PCR)-based analysis and results in maps that are linear orders of DNA sequences along the chromosome. In most cases, markers are anonymous, frequently polymorphic, sequences. These are widely referred to as sequence tag sites (STSs; Olson *et al.*, 1989). These maps are in principle related to the physical or genetic map since some of the markers will be derived from sequences that have themselves independently been positioned on alternative maps. Integration is far from complete. The utility of such maps was underestimated. It was felt that the next level of physical mapping, at the cloned DNA level, would make the recombination/hybrid map level redundant but this has proved not to be the case.

1.3 YAC maps of chromosomes

The size and logistics of working on the whole human genome at the yeast artificial chromosome (YAC) level has meant that all but the CEPH/Genethon consortium have focused upon individual human chromosomes. The construction of YAC-based physical maps of chromosomes has been widely worked upon and reported (Foote *et al.*, 1992; Cohen *et al.*, 1993). The majority of analyses make use of STS content mapping; YACs are arranged into order by virtue of containing the same STS (Fig. 1). In principle, no knowledge of the order of STS is required to generate maps. Order is established at the same time as YAC order is established but this hope has been confounded by two features: all large YAC libraries contain up to 60% of chimeric YACs (chimeras are YACs that contain a piece of DNA that is derived from DNA that is non-contiguous in the human genome, for example a fragment of chromosome 11 joined to a fragment of chromosome 2 DNA). A second problem has been the analysis of unstable YACs. Internal STSs can be missing even though flanking STSs may be present. Both artefacts cause false positives or false negatives and it has not been possible to develop large contigs without prior knowledge of STS order. It was the identification of this set of problems that resulted in a reassessment of the role of recombination and radiation hybrid maps, since these can generate the necessary (large) number of ordered STSs.

STS content mapping has also been used in conjunction with large-scale hybridization analyses. YACs immobilized on filters are probed with individually mapped DNA fragments to generate the hybridization content of a YAC. This can be treated in a formally analogous fashion to STS content. Chromosome 22 (Bentley, personal communication) is a particularly developed example.

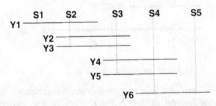

Fig. 1 STS content mapping. Five YACs, Y1–5, are analysed by PCR for the presence or abscence of five STSs, S1–5. Assembling the YACs into overlapping groups by the STSs they contain results not only in the YAC order, but also the STS order, being defined. Note that in practice, the order of S1–5 is established and this eliminates YACs that are chimeric and that consequently contain the 'wrong' STS.

Substantial YAC maps of chromosomes 3, 7, 11, 12, 21, 22, Y and X have been, or are about to be, published (Foote *et al.*, 1992; Green *et al.*, 1994; Kumlien *et al.*, 1994; Nizetic *et al.*, 1994), as well as large whole genome maps developed by the CEPH/Genethon consortium (Cohen *et al.*, 1993).

It is worth pointing out here that a number of areas of research have been part of the HGP but are no longer given much attention: in particular, the construction of large-scale restriction maps of chromosomes was initially thought to be important but there is now widespread acceptance that the information content of such maps, combined with the undoubted technical problems in generating them, enormously reduces the importance of this activity.

1.4 Cosmid maps to genomic sequence

The next step in the programme is the construction of finer detailed cloned DNA maps. These maps have or will have two roles: substrates for gene finding in positional cloning ventures and substrates for large-scale sequencing. Current activities centre around cosmids, since these are currently the only vectors that have proved satisfactory for both purposes (Sulston *et al.*, 1992). However, considerable interest has been shown in both bacterial artificial chromosome (BAC) and P1 vector systems (Shizuya *et al.*, 1992; Pierce *et al.*, 1992), but neither have yet found widespread use in genome projects. Reservations about cloning vectors are discussed below.

Two methods are being employed to construct cosmid-level maps of chromosomes: cosmid binning and fingerprinting. Both have particular advantages.

1.5 Cosmid binning

The principle of this method is shown in Fig. 2: YAC DNAs, stripped of repeat sequences by appropriate pre-hybridization, are hybridized to arrays of cosmids immobilized, as colonies, on filters. Using the appropriate databases, sets of cosmids are defined by each hybridization and these sets will partially overlap if partially overlapping YACs are used as probes. In practice, a minimal tiling path, or slightly redundant minimal tiling path, of YACs is used. This places cosmids into 'bins' defined by the overlapping regions of the YACs (Fig. 2). The smaller the bin, the

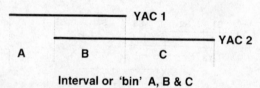

Interval or 'bin' A, B & C

Fig. 2 Cosmid 'binning'. YAC 1 has been used in hybridization experiments to identify cosmid clones. These must necessarily map to the interval, or 'bin' A plus B. YAC 2, in similar analyses, identifies a set of cosmids, some of which are the same as those identified by YAC 1 and some novel. These must map to interval B and C. Clones identified by YACs 1 and 2 must be located in interval B. Thus two YACs define three intervals or bins. This process is normally carried out for a minimal tiling path (the smallest number of YACs that span a region) and therefore the bins are rather large.

higher the resolution of the resulting map. The result of this process has also been referred to as a 'pocket map' (Nizetic *et al.*, 1994). The drawback of binning is that it does not establish true cosmid contigs: the relationship of the hybridizing cosmids is only defined by the bin size and consequently the bins contain unordered cosmids.

It is not yet clear how many YACs need to be analysed to bin cosmids for a whole chromosome.

1.6 Cosmid fingerprinting

The principles of this method were first defined by Coulson *et al.* (1986) and are detailed in Fig. 3. In outline, cosmids, selected at random, are digested with an enzyme (in our case, *Hin*DIII) that generates 8–10 fragments of human DNA on average. The sites are labelled by end-filling with reverse transcriptase, the DNA cut to completion and the fragment analysed on acrylamide sequencing gels. A set of programs based upon those of Sulston's Contig 9 (Sulston *et al.*, 1988, 1989) are then used to digitize the band pattern of each cosmid, normalize the migration distance by reference to marker tracks and store the normalized mobilities. The programs Image and Contig C were developed from those of Sulston *et al.* (1989) to run under UNIX, by R. Durbin and F. Wobus at the Sanger Centre (Hinxton). The cosmid mobilities in the database are then compared pair-wise: overlapping fragment patterns indicate overlapping DNA cloned in the recombinant and this information allows us to construct contigs of cosmids.

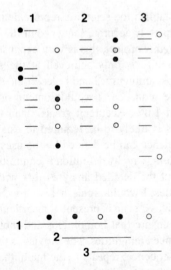

Fig. 3 Fingerprint analysis: three cosmids, 1–3, have been fragmented by the appropriate set of restriction enzymes and the band patterns are shown. The dots mark fragments which are unique to cosmid 1, shared between 1 and 2, shared between 1, 2 and 3, shared between 2 and 3 and finally unique to 3. The lower part of the figure shows the logical relationship between the cosmid that can be deduced from these data. In practice, many thousands of cosmids are analysed independently.

There are cosmid fingerprint projects running on chromosomes 11 (detailed below) and 19. The chromosome 16 project makes use of a blotting protocol to develop fingerprint bands, rather than restriction enzyme digestion (Stallings *et al.*, 1990, 1992), but the logic of the subsequent analysis is identical.

The major advantages of this approach are that actual contigs are constructed and these are a faithful representation of the genome. However, because the analysis is random, it is not possible to get complete contiguity of cosmids covering the whole genome. Additionally, it is clear that cosmids have problems cloning some DNAs, even though it is not clear how extensive this problem actually is in human DNA. This is discussed below.

The contigs that are generated by these analyses can then be sequenced.

2 DNA sequencing

The model for sequencing DNA on a large scale remains the *C. elegans* project: the methods used have been extensively described (Sulston *et al.*, 1992) and it is likely that human DNAs will be sequenced in a similar fashion. Fluorescent sequencing is essentially carried out using random single strand phage shot gun analyses of individual minimal tiling path cosmids and extensive computerized data collection and analysis. The ABI (Applied Biosystems Inc.) sequencers appear to be the universal choice of the large-scale operations.

2.1 What do we want from DNA sequencing?

It is important that we establish the scientific requirements of DNA sequencing. In principle, we want a completely accurate sequence of the whole genome but, as has been shown by the *C. elegans* project, this is very expensive. Sequence accuracy of >99.9% and 100% contiguity is only achieved at the expense of laborious and expensive analysis of gaps, ambiguities and holes in the sequence. The question is, do we need such accurate sequence? I would contend not: the variance of human DNA is between 0.1 and 1.0%. Accuracy greater than this is redundant, since a population-based analysis is likely to be required to establish 'correct' sequences. Thus the accuracy of sequence can be defined by the uses we will put the sequence to: in most cases the end user, who by definition is committed to a full understanding of the gene, will carry out the detailed analyses that will identify polymorphisms and will resolve ambiguities. I would argue that what we require is a sequence that unambiguously demonstrates a gene is present at a particular location, that identifies sufficient of its exons to ensure that homologies and motifs are identified but that may have gaps and sequence ambiguities. The proviso is that we must know the size of gaps and the types of sequence, repeats in the main, that fall into sequence gaps. This type of sequence has been named 'sequence maps' by Sulston and Waterstone (Marshall, 1995). It is an important concept: the sequence map is much cheaper to generate than the complete sequence, simply because the detailed finishing phase is ignored.

3 Alternative approaches

So far, we have discussed the genomic approach to the HGP. Elsewhere in this volume is an extensive discussion of the direct cDNA sequencing approach to the genome and it is clear that this has some powerful arguments, not least cost and speed, in its favour. However, I would argue that cDNA sequencing has the major drawback that it provides only a limited amount of information that relates to only the first of the goals of the HGP, detailed above. There are also theoretical problems of completion of a random sampling of cDNA libraries and the proportion of genes that are expressed in tight developmental (spatial and/or temporal) windows is completely unknown. The map location of sequences is also not established by sequence analysis and this is a major theoretical drawback. The extent of coverage of cDNA sequencing is hard to calculate but there can be little doubt that it is a reasonably cheap approach to the discovery of new genes.

4 The example of chromosome 11

4.1 The biology of chromosome 11

Human chromosome 11 contains 144 Mb of DNA or 4.5% of the genome (Morton, 1991). The entire DNA complement of the chromosome could be contained in 4200 35 kb non-redundant cosmids. The current genetic and physical map of the chromosome has recently been summarized by van Heyningen and Little (1995).

The chromosome is perhaps second only to the X chromosome in the extent of information that has been gathered about it. Over 67 genes, 467 mapped DNA fragments and about 100 chromosomally defined breakpoints have been identified. In addition, a well-characterized monochromosome hybrid, J1, is available and an extensive set of deletion derivatives of this cell line that has facilitated mapping by regional assignment to breakpoint-defined intervals. A set of cosmids that uniquely defines most of these intervals has been derived (Redeker et al., 1994).

An extensive set of 86 radiation hybrids has also been developed from J1 (James et al., 1994) and 506 STS markers positioned on them. Many of these have also been mapped in recombination studies (Gyapay et al., 1994).

YAC mapping of the chromosome is well advanced but not yet published: 650 STSs have been YAC mapped by the CEPH/Genethon consortium, over 900 YACs assembled into more than 100 contigs by Evans (personal communication) and Shows and collaborators (Buffalo, NY) are analysing a further 1800 YACs. In many cases the same YACs have been independently analysed, creating the possibility of data integration.

Pulse field gel electrophoresis (PFGE) maps of >14 Mb from regions of 11p15 and >15 Mb for 11p13/14 have been constructed by Redeker et al. (1994) and Fantes et al. (1995), and extensive maps of 11cen–11q13 and 11q22 regions have also been constructed.

We have carried out a very extensive fingerprint analysis of this chromosome: we have generated 9594 fingerprints, ca 5000 from 11p hybrid cell line-derived cosmids and ca 4500 from a sorted chromosome 11 cosmid library (Smith *et al.*, 1993). These clones are arranged in 1119 contigs with mean occupancy of 3.9 cosmids, mean size 57 kb and maximum size 223 kb.

It is difficult to establish the extent of cosmid coverage of the chromosome, partly because we have used two different sources of clones and partly because random number simulations are not predicative (Coulson and Sulston, personal communication). If we assume that the DNA within the 11p hybrid line is 70% 11p derived (Hoovers *et al.*, 1992) and that 11p is 42% of 11 (Morton, 1991), we can achieve a crude estimate that 5100 clones derive from 11p and 2300 from 11q. This would correspond to about 2.9-fold coverage of 11p and 1-fold coverage of 11q. The calculated Monte Carlo modelling of the current project status would be 1400 contigs with mean length 57 kb and 4.46 occupancy. Our actual progress is slightly less than this and we would guess that this is in part due to non-chromosome 11 regions contained in our original hybrid cell line analyses and to a highly conservative choice of overlaps. The proportion of unclonable regions within chromosome 11 is at present unknown.

5 Unclonable DNAs

Much anecdotal evidence exists that suggests regions of DNA are unclonable in cosmids. Over 90% of *C. elegans* DNA is clonable (Coulson, personal communication) but we have no data relating to human DNA. It has been argued the BAC vectors are more stable than cosmids (Shizuya *et al.*, 1992) but the evidence for this is misleading. BACs are stable to serial propagation whereas cosmids delete and rearrange. The basis for this has been discussed by Little and Cross (1985), but this is not the basis of unclonability in libraries. We do not see large numbers of rearranged cosmids in human libraries or in *C. elegans*. Instead there is a complete absence of some DNAs and this cannot be due to instability (which, at its extreme, would leave empty vectors). Unclonability appears to be associated with an inability of the insert DNA to enter the *E. coli* cell: there is no obvious physical explanation for this phenomenon. The effect of this is that there will be real gaps in the cosmid coverage. Thus we have unclonable gaps ('holes') and random sampling 'gaps' in coverage. How are these dealt with in the sequence map approach?

5.1 Ordering of contigs prior to sequencing—the importance of resource sharing

The best illustration of the methods used for ordering contigs is given by the example of the international chromosome 11 project. We have estimated above that there will be about 1000–1500 gaps and holes in our cosmid map after the fingerprinting programme has finished: many of the gaps will be imaginary (overlapping by too small an amount to allow fingerprint assembly) or reasonably small.

Binning analysis, carried out by a number of laboratories, uses the chromosome

11 cosmid arrays as targets: since we are systematically fingerprinting this library, our contigs will attach themselves to bins. All that is required to achieve this is a measure of data exchange and this is set in place by international collaborations (Zehetner and Lehrach, 1994). The main international approach, and our own laboratory, uses a minimal tiling path of YAC clones that represent the best YAC map of chromosome 11. Each minimal tiling path clone is used to make AluPCR-based probes and hybridized to our cosmid libraries (AluPCR is a strategy for producing specific DNA probes from genomic DNA by priming PCR reactions from flanking highly repetitive Alu repeat elements). A proportion of cosmids corresponding to the YAC will be hit: it does not have to be 100%, since a high proportion of the cosmids will be in contigs. This will link contig to YAC, to map. We can only crudely estimate the number of minimal tiling path clones. If CEPH (Centre d'Etude Polymorphisme Humain) megaYACs were exclusively used, it would be perhaps 300 (the chimerism of these YACs would not be a problem since the target cosmids are all chromosome 11 derived). Through our own analyses and collaborations we have already positioned over 400 of our contigs and thus some ordering is already established.

What we hope to achieve by these and similar protocols, are contigs that are ordered with respect to the YAC bins. Sizes of holes and gaps can be directly determined. It is likely that some amount of work will still be required to position individual contigs within bins, but this can be carried out quite late in the programme.

6 Computer data

A key component of this collaborative approach is to have data exchange mechanisms. In part this is achieved by resource sharing of filters and libraries but it will also require the development of extensive computer tools. We are developing such tools based upon the ACEDB database of Durbin and Thierry-Mieg. It is fair to say that this is a considerable undertaking: data analyses are rarely complete, i.e. the same clone analysed with respect to the same mapping tools (breakpoints, YACs, cosmids, cell lines etc.) and thus data can be formally incapable of integrated presentation. Multiple displays of data, mapping to different representations of the chromosome, is the best that can be hoped for until a more complete, YAC- and cosmid-based, analysis supplants these more crude mapping reagents.

7 Conclusion

The generation of large-scale maps and sequences from the genome of humans is technically possible. Maps and sequences will not be complete, but order will be established and the biological application of these partial analyses will be as profound in its impact as if the sequences and maps were complete. The important point is that sequence maps of all human chromosomes are an achievable goal by the millennium: similar analyses can then be carried out for the mouse and the other human genetic surrogates. This is the important development of the sequence map concept.

Acknowledgements

I would like to thank members of my laboratory, including Scott Ellis, Ben Arnold, Mark Strivens, Andy Ryan and Aviva Ward. I am indebted to many colleagues but in particular would like to thank Veronica van Heyningen, Wendy Bickmore, Marcel Mannens, Jan Hoovers and Glen Evans. Work reported in this paper was supported by the Human Genome Project directed programme of the MRC, by the CRC, and by grants from the EC.

References

Cohen, D., Chumakov, I. and Weissenbach, J. (1993). *Nature* **366**, 698–701.

Coulson, A., Sulston, J., Brenner, S. and Karn, J. (1986). *Proc. Natl. Acad. Sci. USA* **83**, 7821–7825.

Fantes, J. A., Oghene, K., Boyle, S., Danes, S., Fletcher, J. M., Bruford, E., Williamson, K., Seawright, A., Schedl, A., Hanson, I. M., Zehetner, G., Bhogal, R., Lehrach, H., Gregory, S., Williams, J., Little, P. F. R., Sellar, G. C., Hoovers, J., Mannens, M., Weissenbach, J., Junien, C., van Heyningen, V. and Bickmore, W. A. (1995). *Genomics* **25**, 447–461.

Foote, S., Vollrath, D., Hilton, A. and Page, D. C. (1992). *Science* **258**, 60–66.

Green, E. D., Idol, J. R., Mohr Tidwell, R. M., Braden, V. V., Peluso, D. C., Fulton, R. S., Massa, H. F., Magness, C. L., Wilson, A. M., Kimura, J., *et al.* (1994). *Hum. Mol. Genet.* **3**, 489–501.

Gyapay, G., Morissette, J., Vignal, A., Dib, C., Fizames, C., Millasseau, P., Marc, S., Bernadi, G., Lathrop, M. and Weissenbach, J. (1994). *Nature Genet.* **7**, 246–339.

Hoovers, J. M. N., Mannens, M., John, R., Bliek, J., van Heyningen, V., Porteous, D. J., Leschot, N. J., Westerwald, A. and Little, P. F. R. (1992). *Genomics* **10**, 254–263.

James, M. R., Richard, C., W-III, Schott, J-J., Yousry, C., Clark, K., Bell, J., Terwilliger, J. D., Hazan, J., Dubay, C., Vignal, A., Agrapart, M., Imai, T., Nakamura, Y., Polymeropoulos, M., Weissenbach, J., Cox, D.R. and Lathrop, G. M. (1994). *Nature Genet.* **8**, 70–76.

Kumlien, J., Labella, T., Zehetner, G., Vatcheva, R., Nizetic D. and Lehrach, H. (1994). *Mamm. Genome* **5**, 365–371.

Little, P. F. R. and Cross, S. H. (1985). *Proc. Natl. Acad. Sci. USA* **82**, 3159–3163.

Marshall, E. (1995). *Science* **267**, 783–784.

Morton, N. E. (1991). *Proc. Natl. Acad. Sci. USA* **88**, 7474–7476.

Nizetic, D., Gellen, L., Hamvas, R. M., Mott, R., Grigoriev, A., Vatcheva, R., Zehetner, G., Yaspo, M.L., Dutriaux, A., Lopes, C., *et al.*, (1994). *Hum. Mol. Genet.* **3**, 759–770.

Olson, M., Hood, L., Cantor, C. and Botstein, D. (1989). *Science* **245**, 1434–1435.

Pierce, J. C., Sternberg, N. and Sauer, B. (1992). *Mamm. Genome* **3**, 550–558.

Redeker, B., Hoovers, J. M., Alders, M., van Moorsel, J. A., Ivens, A. C., Gregory, S., Bliek, J., de Galan, L., van den Bogaard, R., Visser, J., van der Voort, R., Feinberg, A. P., Little, P. F. R., Westerwald, A. and Mannens, M. (1994). *Genomics* **21**, 538–550.

Shizuya, H., Birren, B., Kim, U. J., Mancino, V., Slepak, T., Tachiiri, Y. and Simon, M. (1992). *Proc. Natl. Acad. Sci. USA* **89**, 8794–8797.

Smith, M. W., Clark, S. P., Hutchinson, J. S., Wei, Y. H., Churukian, A. C., Daniels, L. B., Diggle, K. L., Gen, M. W., Romo, A. J, Lin, Y, Selleri, L., McElligott, D. L. and Evans, G. A. (1993). *Genomics* **17**, 699–725.

Stallings, R. L., Torney, D. C., Hildebrand, C. E., Longmire, J. L., Deaven, L. L. and Jett, J. H., Doggett, N. A. and Moyzis, R. K. (1990). *Proc. Natl. Acad. Sci. USA* **87**, 6218–6222.

Stallings, R. L., Doggett, N. A., Callen, D., Apostolou S., Chen, L. Z., Nancarrow, J. K., Whitmore, S. A., Harris, P., Michison, H., Breuning, M. *et al.* (1992). *Genomics* **13**, 1031–1039.

Sulston, J., Mallett, F., Staden, R., Durbin R., Horsnell, T. and Coulson, A. (1988). *Comput. Appl. Biosci.* **4**, 125–132.

Sulston, J., Mallett F., Durbin R. and Horsnell T. (1989). *Comput. Appl. Biosci.* **5**, 101–106.

Sulston, J., Du Z., Thomas, K., Wilson, R., Hillier, L., Staden, R., Halloran, N., Green, P., Thierry-Mieg, J., Qiu L. *et al.,* (1992). *Nature* **356**, 37–41.

van Heyningen, V. and Little, P. F. R. (1995). *Cytogenet. Cell Genet.* **69**, (in press).

Weissenbach, J., Gyapay G., Dib, C., Vignal, A., Morissette, J., Millasseau, P., Vaysseix, G. and Lathrop, M. (1992). *Nature* **359**, 794–801.

Zehetner, G. and Lehrach, H. (1994). *Nature* **367**, 489–491.

2

Progress Towards a Complete Set of Human Genes

MARK D. ADAMS

The Institute for Genomic Research, 9712 Medical Center Drive, Rockville, MD20850, USA

Abstract

A major goal of the human genome project is identification of the complete set of human genes. Single-pass, partial sequencing of cDNA clones to generate expressed sequence tags (ESTs) provides a rapid method of gene discovery (Adams *et al.*, 1991), which has been widely applied in humans and other species. The EST strategy was developed to permit rapid identification of expressed genes by sequence analysis, while at the same time providing a key resource for gene mapping (Adams *et al.*, 1991; Polymeropoulos *et al.*, 1993). The Institute for Genomic Research (TIGR) has sequenced ESTs from over 300 human cDNA libraries made from single cells, fetal and embryonic tissues, a large number of adult organs and tissues, and cancerous tissues. The combination of data on gene expression and putative gene functions inferred from sequence similarity provides a powerful means of assessing the transcriptional activity of the genome in the cells and tissues of an organism.

As more EST sequences are obtained, we have been able to assemble the ESTs into contigs. Elimination of sequence redundancy resulted in identification of over 40 000 distinct, non-overlapping cDNA sequences. The contigs also allow an analysis of the tissue distribution of expression of the transcript by analysis of the libraries from which the ESTs were derived.

Several EST studies are under way based upon the premise that most physiological and pathological conditions will result in or from a change in the gene expression patterns of cells and tissues. A study evaluating differences in expression with nerve growth factor treatment of rat PC12 cells identified several hundred differentially regulated transcripts (Lee *et al.*, 1995). Quantitative changes in gene expression identified by EST sampling were confirmed for several genes by Northern analysis. Prior to high throughput DNA and EST sequencing, such studies would not have been possible.

GENOMES, MOLECULAR BIOLOGY AND DRUG DISCOVERY
ISBN 0-12-137790-3

TIGR has established the Human cDNA Database (HCD) to provide researchers at non-profit institutions access to cDNA/EST sequence and related data from TIGR and Human Genome Sciences (HGS). HCD functions as an 'e-mail server'. The data in HCD will initially include approximately 90 000 sequences obtained at TIGR along with approximately 60 000 sequences from HGS that have significant overlap with TIGR sequences or sequences in the public domain. These sequences represent between 30 000 and 35 000 unique human genes.

1 Introduction

Expressed sequence tags (ESTs) were introduced in 1991 as a means of rapidly characterizing genes expressed in the human brain (Adams et al., 1991). Investigators in fields as diverse as human genetic diseases (Papadopoulos et al., 1994; Dodt et al., 1995) and plant physiology (Newman et al., 1994) have found that the EST methodology can provide an inexpensive and rapid first glimpse at the genes expressed in a certain tissue or under a certain set of conditions. Because of its relative simplicity, the EST approach to genome characterization has been adopted in many countries with modest biology and genome budgets and in developing countries as a practical way both to import state-of-the-art technology and to participate in genome studies of organisms of local relevance, such as Schistosoma mansoni (Franco et al., 1995) and the filarial parasites (M. Blaxter, personal communication).

2 EST sequencing at The Institute for Genomic Research

The laboratory aspects of EST sequencing are quite straightforward (Fig. 1); it is the information management—sequence analysis and comparative studies—which is complex and potentially open-ended. An EST project begins with an experimental question to answer such as: 'what genes are expressed in liver?' or 'what are the differences in expression between normal and transformed cells?' or 'what are the most abundantly expressed genes in this species?' Selection of tissue samples for preparation of mRNA is driven by these questions.

Construction of a representative cDNA library is critical so that the distribution of EST sequences can be assumed reliably to reflect the steady-state mRNA levels in the tissue from which the library was made. cDNA library construction has been reviewed previously (Moreno-Planques and Fuldner, 1994). Over 300 cDNA libraries were constructed for the EST sequencing projects at The Institute for Genomic Research (TIGR) (Adams et al., 1995). The majority of these libraries were constructed using the lambdaZAP phage system (Stratagene, La Jolla, CA). Wherever possible, quality control checks should be built into the procedure to assess the yield, determine whether amplification alters the proportion of non-recombinant or marker clones etc. An extensive quality control regimen was developed to assess the quality of each library prior to and during large-scale sequencing (Table 1). Over half of the libraries were rejected or remade due to skewed

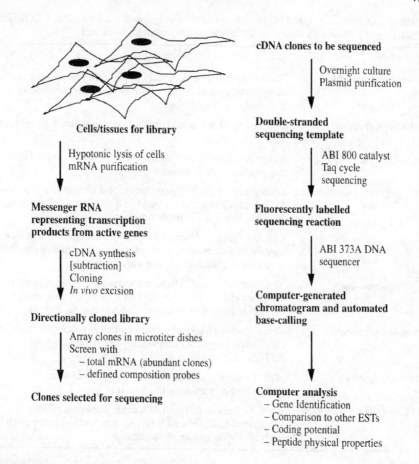

Fig. 1 Flow diagram for an EST project. The building blocks of an EST project are listed with key decision points. At each step, relevant lab techniques including mRNA purification, cDNA library construction, clone selection, and automated sequencing are shown. Many variations on this theme are possible, depending upon the specific application, such as subtraction or screening of the library to bias sequencing toward particular groups of clones. Computational analysis may also take many forms based around sequence similarity searching and compositional characteristics.

representation of transcripts, unacceptably high levels of non-recombinant clones or mitochondrial transcripts, or small insert sizes. Several libraries contained large numbers of clones for a few very abundant mRNA species, reflecting high levels of expression of certain genes. While these libraries were representative, they were not suited to large-scale sequencing. Libraries with highly abundant cDNAs were screened with total cDNA or specific clones in order to increase the diversity of clones sequenced. Nearly all libraries were directionally cloned, meaning that the polyA tail of the mRNA is cloned adjacent to a specific end of the vector. Directional cloning allows a choice of 5′ vs 3′ ends for sequencing.

Table 1 Quality control and evaluation. Quality control procedures for each step in the EST process are listed with specific points of evaluation or standards to be met

Procedure	Quality control and evaluation
Tissue procurement	Tissues snap frozen as quickly as possible post-mortem; tissue samples that tested positive for HIV and/or hepatitis were not used
mRNA purification	500 μg total RNA to start; mRNA concentration determined by spot blot
cDNA synthesis	Tracer levels of ^{32}P included; agarose gel examination for degradation; size selection > 500 bp
cDNA library construction	Blue/white screen for inserts before and after *in vivo* excision; PCR to check insert size—must be 1.0–1.5kb average; libraries must contain > 0.5×10^6 recombinants
Sample sequencing	Check gene diversity and content, mitochondrial contamination, insert size, % full length, Alu (highly repeated sequence in human DNA) content, directionality
Library screening	Screening with total cDNA, mitochondrial genome, or specific abundant cDNA clones; rechecked by sample sequencing to confirm reduction of abundant cDNAs (also see Fig. 1)
Template preparation	Concentration checked by CytoFluor or agarose gels; some sets checked by sample sequencing; clone location tracking in ESTDB; success rate tracked in ESTDB
DNA sequencing	pGEM control plasmids on ~1/4 of sequencer runs; protocol/reagent tracking in ESTDB
EST sequence quality check	< 3% Ns (base in DNA sequence that cannot be reliably assigned as A, C, G or T) > 100 bp; matches to known genes; analysis of non-human contamination

The primary decision point in EST sequencing is whether to sequence 5′ ends, 3′ ends, or both. Especially in mammalian mRNA, the 3′ untranslated sequence can be quite long (e.g. 2.4 kb in the obesity gene (Zhang *et al.,* 1994)). Since protein-coding information is most useful for gene identification, 5′ ends are preferred for gene discovery applications. 3′ ends provide much more robust analysis of redundancy for comparative projects since cDNAs representing transcripts from the same gene can always be grouped accurately (assuming no gross differences in polyadenylation site). Choosing to sequence both ends of clones answers both goals, but at a reduction in throughput since two reactions are done on each clone rather than one. We have used a combination of approaches, depending on the project. Frequently, clones are selected for sequencing from both ends based on the results of gene identification and grouping, thus minimizing the number of additional sequencing reactions which must be performed.

For the EST sequencing, plasmid templates (prepared using a procedure from AGTC, Inc., Gaithersburg, MD) were reacted using fluorescent dye-labelled sequencing primers and cycle sequencing with *Taq* polymerase. Reactions were run on Applied Biosystems 373 DNA Sequencers. The large volume of materials and information that is handled in a project of this scale requires careful attention to standards of quality and quality control to ensure that the resulting sequences will meet minimum standards of accuracy (Adams *et al.*, 1994). A laboratory information management system has been developed based around the Sybase relational database management system (ESTDB; Kerlavage *et al.*, 1993). Software was written to pass information on template preparation, sequencing reactions, and sequencing gel runs to ESTDB. This system provides the basis for tracking ongoing projects and maintaining quality control. Accurate management of projects is the beginning of sequence analysis. All ESTs are subjected to an initial standard sequence analysis protocol. This includes identification of repetitive elements, classification of matches to known human genes, searches against the public protein and nucleic acid databases, comparison with other ESTs, and assessment of potential to contain a protein-coding region. For an average library, between 30% and 50% of the ESTs can be putatively identified based on sequence similarity to a gene from human or other organism. The remainder remain unidentifiable, but substantial information can still be derived by examining the cDNA libraries in which they were found.

cDNA libraries generally reflect the mRNA abundance in the tissue from which they are made. Therefore, more ESTs are obtained from abundantly expressed transcripts than from rare transcripts. Correct association of ESTs and genes is essential to calculate redundancy and accurately assess the distribution of expression of genes in different tissues. For ESTs matching known human genes, this process is reasonably straightforward, because even non-overlapping ESTs can be assigned to the same gene unambiguously by a match to the complete sequence from GenBank. To facilitate the association of ESTs with known human genes, we developed a canonical set of human cDNA sequences from GenBank (HT sequences; Adams *et al.*, 1995). The HT dataset contains a non-redundant set of human genes with associated annotation such as coding regions, splice isoforms, and exon–intron boundaries. For each sequence in the HT dataset, a profile of gene expression was constructed indicating the relative level of expression of that gene in each cDNA library studied.

ESTs that do not exactly match a sequence in GenBank are more difficult to analyse in terms of redundancy and distribution. To identify the degree of redundancy and build sets of overlapping ESTs, software was developed to build assemblies of ESTs. These contigs were named tentative human consensus sequences (THCs). The THC assembly software was designed to minimize the contribution of alternatively spliced or chimeric ESTs. If an individual EST had a region of mismatch with the consensus sequence, it was excluded from the assembly. This resulted in construction of separate assemblies for different splice isoforms. THCs were evaluated using the process described above for ESTs. Over 70% of the THCs have no match to sequences in the public databases. Examination of the tissue distribution of THCs revealed several abundant clones that were apparently

Table 2 Tissue-specific and widely expressed novel genes. Example THCs matched by at least 10 ESTs from a single tissue, but not from any other tissues, are listed as potentially tissue-specific, abundant genes. Also listed are two novel THCs containing ESTs from at least 20 of the 30 tissues from which more than 1000 ESTs were obtained.

THC No.	Number of ESTs	Tissue
31361	26	Testis
9969	14	Brain
9214	11	Brain
11971	12	Brain
16933	13	White blood cells
11412	99	Many
11406	72	Many

tissue-specific or widely expressed and do not match any previously known gene (Table 2).

3 Comparative gene anatomy

EST sequencing has been used as a comparative tool in several projects. One comparative project at TIGR has been to examine changes in gene expression with nerve growth factor (NGF) treatment of the rat pheochromocytoma cell line PC12 (Greene and Tischler, 1982; Halegoua *et al.*, 1991). Pheochromocytoma is a tumour of the adrenal gland. PC12 cells are neuronal in origin; when grown in the absence of NGF, their morphology is round and they divide regularly. After 3 days treatment with NGF they terminally differentiate, going into mitotic arrest and developing neuritic outgrowths. PC12 cells have been studied extensively as a model of differentiation and as a model of cellular change with drug treatment. Previous studies of gene expression in these cells had identified fewer than 12 differentially expressed genes.

About 3500 ESTs were obtained from cDNA libraries made from untreated and NGF-treated (9 days) PC12 cells (Lee *et al.*, 1995). Through analysis of the genes matched by ESTs and grouping overlapping ESTs into assemblies representing distinct genes, several hundred genes that are potentially up- or down-regulated with NGF treatment were identified. To confirm that the libraries were in fact representative of the steady-state mRNA levels, several ESTs which appeared more frequently in one library than the other were used to probe Northern blots of total RNA from untreated and NGF-treated PC12 cells. A statistically significant correlation was found between EST levels and steady-state mRNA levels. Examples of genes with altered expression are shown in Table 3. Generally speaking, several genes indicative of the neuronal phenotype were apparently up-regulated; several genes associated with replication and passage through the cell cycle were apparently

Table 3 Genes up- or down-regulated by NGF in PC12 cells

Gene	% ESTs in control	% ESTs in NGF-treated
Proliferation-associated gene	0.40	0.18
Chromogranin A	0.25	0.03
Glutaminyl-tRNA synthetase	0.15	0
MAP kinase kinase	0.1	0
Cu-Zn superoxide dismutase	0	0.15
Clusterin	0	0.14
Neurofilament L chain	0	0.08

down-regulated. Interestingly, a large number of genes without database matches were also found more frequently in one library than the other. This demonstrates that EST analysis can be used, with properly constructed cDNA libraries, to assess broad-based changes in gene expression.

4 An expression map of the human genome

A demonstration of the power of EST sequencing to discover new genes involved in disease is the identification of three new genes that are mutated in inherited forms of colon cancer. Colon and other cancers are characterized at the molecular level by an accumulation of mutations in the DNA of transformed cells, including expansion of di- and trinucleotide repeats. Because of these defects, it was proposed that DNA repair enzymes may be altered or missing in cancerous cells. One gene, called *hMSH2*, was cloned (Leach *et al.*, 1993; Fishel *et al.*, 1993) based on sequence similarity to yeast and *Escherichia coli* DNA repair enzymes. Mutations in this gene were shown to segregate with affected members of families exhibiting hereditary non-polyposis colon cancer (HNPCC), thereby demonstrating that the DNA repair defect is likely a cause rather than an effect of transformation. Because the DNA repair pathways in bacteria and yeast are complex and involve many enzymes, it was hypothesized that additional human repair enzyme genes might exist. Searches of TIGR's EST database with bacterial and yeast DNA repair enzyme protein sequences revealed three additional genes, each with striking similarity to the bacterial and yeast enzymes. Each new gene was mapped and determined to be in a chromosomal region associated with HNPCC. Full-length sequencing of the coding region of the genes and comparison of the sequence from normal and affected individuals resulted in identification of mutations in each gene which associated with the disease in affected families (Papadopoulos *et al.*, 1994; Nicolaides *et al.*, 1994). The ability to screen individuals who are at risk of developing HNPCC either to eliminate them as carriers of the disease genes or to identify them for more careful observation will be a dramatic improvement in pre-symptomatic treatment of HNPCC.

In the case of the HNPCC genes, the search for candidate genes was driven by a hypothesis about the involvement of DNA repair enzymes. The candidate genes were straightforward to identify based on a similarity search of the database; additional weight was given to these genes as candidates by mapping them to regions implicated in disease. For many inherited disorders, however, no clues to the biological mechanism exist, and the only starting point is to try to identify all candidate genes within a chromosomal interval defined by the closest genetically linked markers.

By the end of 1995, it is likely that several hundred thousand human ESTs will have been sequenced throughout the world and placed in publicly accessible databases. The gene discovery aspect of EST analysis is therefore well along, with most genes represented by multiple ESTs. The next phase of application of ESTs to genome characterization is assignment of ESTs to unique chromosomal locations. This serves to pinpoint the location of the gene matched by the EST and builds a bridge between the current physical maps of the genome and the genes themselves. The map of ESTs is called an 'expression map' because it combines information on gene locations and expression patterns.

An expression map should prove useful in several areas of genome research, but none more so than in inherited disease identification. The current process of positional cloning is quite laborious. After demonstration of linkage of a disease in families with a particular genetic marker (and thus chromosomal location), positional cloning involves isolation of the physical DNA containing the chromosomal region of interest (e.g. a clone from the physical map) followed by attempts to identify the genes within the region. Once these candidate genes have been identified, they can be screened for mutations in patients inheriting the disease. Candidate gene identification can be approached in many ways, including complete sequencing, cDNA selection (Lovett *et al.*, 1991), and exon amplification (Buckler *et al.*, 1991). A saturated expression map, one with all of the genes localized, would eliminate the need for all of these gene-finding techniques. A partial map, one with only some genes, will provide an immediate set of candidate genes to be evaluated for mutations while other techniques are initiated. The recent description of cloning of the breast cancer gene resulted from an extensive effort to identify all possible candidate genes (Miki *et al.*, 1994).

The current genetic and physical maps of the human genome (Cohen *et al.*, 1993; Murray *et al.*, 1994) are based on non-gene markers such as simple sequence repeats and randomly isolated sequence tag sites (STSs). Genetic maps are, by definition, ordered because they represent recombination frequencies between polymorphic sites. Polymorphic STSs can be used as anchor points in construction of a physical map. In the case of the CEPH yeast artificial chromosome (YAC) map, YACs corresponding to 2000 polymorphic STSs were identified; these formed the skeleton on which the map was built. Other methods of identifying overlapping YACs were used to build bridges between the YACs containing polymorphic STSs. In this way, a map covering approximately 70% of the genome was constructed (Cohen *et al.*, 1993). There is thus about a 70% chance of being able to map an EST to a CEPH YAC of known location. The YAC location provides information on chromosome location and a physically cloned piece of DNA for further manipulation in disease gene discovery.

Another form of physical map is called a 'statistical radiation hybrid map'. Radiation hybrids are formed by irradiating human DNA to break it into small pieces of DNA from 100 kb to several megabases in size (Cox, 1992). The human DNA is transformed into a rodent cell line, where it is stably maintained. Each human–rodent somatic cell hybrid contains about 20% of the human genome in hundreds of small pieces. In an analogous way to construction of the YAC map, a series of markers is used to 'type' each hybrid cell line to develop a profile of the chromosomal fragments it carries. Once this profile is developed, the location of an unknown marker can be determined by comparison of its profile with those of the known markers. The map is 'statistical' in the sense that profiles will rarely be exact matches; discrepancies increase with the distance between the location of the unknown marker and the nearest anchor point. A series of well-spaced anchor markers with known order and cytogenetic location is therefore essential for the utility of radiation hybrids.

Different approaches to disease gene discovery require different materials and different methodologies, dependent upon the particular circumstances. For instance, if the location of a disease gene has been genetically defined to a small region of chromosome 4, then the location of ESTs on a radiation hybrid map is sufficient to define candidate genes. If the goal is to obtain the complete genomic sequence of a region or to use other gene-finding techniques such as cDNA selection (Lovett *et al.,* 1991) or exon amplification (Buckler *et al.,* 1991), the cloned DNA, such as obtained from the YAC map, is necessary.

For several (sometimes contradictory) maps to be useful, they need to be integrated (correlated to one another along their lengths) so that a position on one can be related to the others. The polymorphic STS-defined genetic markers have proven a useful tool for map integration since they have been placed on both the YAC and radiation hybrid maps. Placement of ESTs on both radiation hybrid and YAC maps will also serve to relate the two to one another. Location of ESTs on both radiation hybrid and YAC maps will also serve to provide candidate gene identification from both entry points to the physical map. Polymorphic STSs and ESTs are likely to become the standard for integrating various types of physical maps. Also, as maps become more precise, the density of markers required increases. For instance, a 10 Mb map of the genome requires only about 400 markers, but a 100 kb map would require 80 000 markers. It would be tremendously useful if these thousands of markers were in fact genes in order to facilitate positional cloning and map construction. A variety of evidence suggests that genes are not uniformly distributed along the genome. Use of ESTs to build physical maps will result in the best map quality in regions of high gene density.

5 Using ESTs in tomorrow's research

The EST methodology has caused a dramatic shift in type and volume of data that is submitted to GenBank. In 1994, over half of the new sequences in GenBank were ESTs. ESTs now represent more than one-third of all sequences in GenBank.

GenBank's EST database dbEST (Boguski *et al.,* 1993) contained over 138 000 sequences as of mid-March 1995. Although more than half of the ESTs in dbEST are from humans, dbEST also contains ESTs from 32 other species. Advances in the automated sequencing technology used by many EST-sequencing laboratories has resulted in improvements over the last several years in the accuracy of single-pass sequences. In general, though, ESTs have a higher error rate, particularly frameshift-causing insertion and deletion errors, than other sequences in GenBank. This can result in missed matches in similarity searches and difficulty in interpreting weak matches (for instance across large phylogenetic distances). Additionally, a substantial redundancy of ESTs from some of the more abundantly expressed human genes are accumulating in GenBank. There are currently over 700 ESTs representing gamma globulin alone. This redundancy can obscure matches to the full-length gene sequence, but more importantly the large number of exact matches returned in some searches can make it more difficult to find the potentially more interesting non-exact matches that define a new member of a gene family.

Dealing with redundancy, variable accuracy, and large amounts of gene identification and sequence data may seem daunting enough; add in (possibly conflicting) mapping data from one or several sources and the EST information explosion seems completely beyond redemption. The National Centre for Biotechnology Information's (NCBI) dbEST is a first attempt to deal with the unique data management requirements of a large volume of ESTs. By establishing dbEST, NCBI has segregated ESTs as a separate division of GenBank which makes them easier to work with. dbEST itself is available on-line in a parsable format to facilitate extracting the information it contains. The next generation of EST databases will address redundancy by representing EST assemblies (e.g. as described above) and the tissue and expression information that can be derived from that redundancy. The truly integrated databases that will ultimately serve researchers in many fields will present sequence, annotation/identification, expression, and mapping information for *genes* rather than ESTs.

6   The Institute for Genomic Research Database

TIGR has established a mechanism for making the EST data available to scientists at non-profit institutions. The TIGR Database (TDB) operates as a World Wide Web server and as an electronic mail server. The goal of the database is to provide broad distribution of the data for research purposes. More information about the database can be obtained by e-mail on info@hcd.tigr.org.

References

Adams, M. D., Kelley, J. M., Gocayne, J. D., Dubnick, M., Polymeropoulos, M. H., Xiao, H., Merril, C. R., Wu, A., Olde, B., Moreno, R. F., Kerlavage, A. R., McCombie, W. R. and Venter, J. C. (1991). *Science* **252**, 1651–1656.
Adams, M. D., Kerlavage, A. R., Kelley, J. M., Gocayne, J. D., Fields, C., Fraser, C. M. and Venter, J. C. (1994). *Nature* **368**, 474–475.

Adams, M. D., Kerlavage, A. R., Fleischmann, R. D. et al. (1995). Initial assessment of human gene diversity and expression patterns based upon 83 million nucleotides of cDNA sequence. Nature 377, (Suppl.), 3–174.

Boguski, M., Lowe, T., and Tolstochev, C. (1993). Nature Genet. 4, 332–333.

Buckler, A. J., Chang, D. D., Graw, S. L., Brook, J. D., Haber, D. A., Sharp, P. A. and Housman, D. E. (1991). Proc. Natl. Acad. Sci. USA 88, 4005–4009.

Cohen, D., Chumakov, I. and Weissenbach, J. (1993). Nature 366, 698–701.

Cox, D. (1992). Cytogenet. Cell Genet. 59, 80–81.

Dodt, G., Braverman, N., Wong, C., Moser, A., Moser, H. W., Watkins, P., Valle, D. and Gould, S. J. (1995). Nature Genet. 9, 115–125.

Fishel, R., Lescoe, M. K., Rao, M. R. S., Copeland, N. G., Jenkins, N. A., Garber, J., Kane, M. and Kolodner, R. (1993). Cell 75, 1027–1038.

Franco, G. R., Adams, M. D., Soares, M. B., Simpson, A. J. G., Venter, J. C. and Pena, S. D. J. (1995). Gene, 152(2), 141–147.

Greene, L. A. and Tischler, A. S. (1982). Adv. Cell. Neurobiol. 3, 373–415.

Halegoua, S., Armstrong, R. C. and Kremer, N. E. (1991). Curr. Top. Microbiol. Immunol. 165, 119–170.

Kerlavage, A. R., Adams, M. D., Kelley, J. C., Dubnick, M., Powell, J., Shanmugam, P., Venter, J. C. and Fields, C. (1993). In Proceedings 26th Hawaii Int. Conf. on System Sciences, pp. I:585–590. IEEE Computer Society Press, Los Alamitos, CA.

Leach, F. S., Nicolaides, N. C., Papadopoulos, N., Liu, B., Jen, J., Parsons, R., Peltomaki, P., Sistonen, P., Aaltonen, L. A., Nystrom-Lahti, M., Guan, X.-Y. Zhang, J., Meltzer, P. S., Yu, J.-W., Kao, F.-T., Chen, D. J., Cerosaletti, K. M., Fournier, R. E. K., Todd, S., Lewis, T., Leach, R. J., Naylor, S. L., Weissenbach, J., Mecklin, J.-P., Jarvinen, H., Petersen, G. M., Hamilton, S. R., Green, J., Jass, J., Watson, P., Lynch, H. T., Trent, J. M. de la Chapelle, A., Kinzler, K. W. and Vogelstein, B. (1993). Cell 75, 1215–1225.

Lee, N. H., Weinstock, K. G., Kirkness, E. F., Earle-Hughes, J. A., Fleischmann, R. D., Fuldner, R. A., Marmaros, S., Glodek, A., Gocayne, J. D., Adams, M. D., Kerlavage, A. R., Fraser, C. M. and Venter, J. C. (1995). Proc. Natl. Acad. Sci. USA 92, 8303–8307.

Lovett, M., Kere, J. and Hinton, L. M. (1991). Proc. Natl. Acad. Sci. USA 88, 9628–9632.

Miki, Y., Swensen, J., Shattuck-Eidens, D., Futreal, P. A., Harshman, K., Tavtigian, S., Liu, Q., Cochran, C., Bennett, L. M., Ding, W., Bell, R., Rosenthal, J., Hussey, C., Tran, T., McClure, M., Frye, C., Hattier, T., Phelps, R., Haugen-Strano, A., Katcher, H., Yakumo, K., Gholami, Z., Shafffer, D., Stone, S., Bayer, S., Wray, C., Bogden, R., Dayananth, P., Ward, J., Tonin, P., Narod, S., Bristow, P. K., Norris, F. H., Helvering, L., Morrison, P., Rosteck, P., Lai, M., Barrett, J. C., Lewis, C., Neuhausen, S., Cannon-Albright, L., Goldgar, D., Wiseman, R., Kamb, A. and Skolnick, M. H. (1994). Science 266, 66–71.

Moreno-Planques, R. F. and Fuldner, R.A. (1994). In Automated DNA Sequencing and Analysis (M. D. Adams, C. Fields and J. C. Venter, eds), pp. 102–108. Academic Press, London.

Murray, J. C., Buetow, K. H., Weber, J. L., Ludwigsen, S., Scherpbier-Heddema, T., Manion, F., Quillen, J., Sheffield, V. C., Sunden, S., Duyk, G. M., Weissenbach, J., Gyapay, Gabor, Dib, C., Morrissette, J., Lathrop, G. M., Vignal, A., White, R., Matsunami, N., Gerken, S., Melis, R., Albertsen, H., Plaetke, R., Odelberg, S., Ward, D., Dausset, J., Cohen, D. and Cann, H. (1994). Science 265, 2049–2054.

Newman, T., de Bruijn, F. J., Green, P., Keegstra, K., Kende, H., McIntosh, L., Ohlrogge, J., Raikhel, N., Somerville, S., Thomashow, M., Retzel, E. and Somerville, C. (1994). Plant Physiol. 106, 1241–1255.

Nicolaides, N. C., Papadopoulos, N., Ruben, S. R., Carter, K. C., Rosen, C. A., Haseltine, W. A., Fleischmann, R. D., Fraser, C. M., Adams, M. D., Venter, J. C., Dunlop, M., Hamilton,

S. R., Peterson, G. M., de la Chapelle, A., Vogelstein, B. and Kinzler, K. W. (1994). *Nature* **371**, 75–80.

Papadopoulos, N., Nicolaides, N. C., Wei, Y-F., Ruben, S. R., Carter, K. C., Rosen, C. A., Haseltine, W. A., Fleischmann, R. D., Fraser, C. M., Adams, M. D., Venter, J. C., Hamilton, S. R., Peterson, G. M., Watson, P., Lynch, H. T., Peltomäke, P., Mecklin, J.-P., de la Chapelle, A., Kinzler, K. W. and Vogelstein, B. (1994). *Science* **263**, 1625–1629.

Polymeropoulos, M. H., Xiao, H., Torres, R., Sikela, J., Adams, M., Venter, J. C. and Merril, C. R. (1993). *Nature Genet.* **4**, 381–386 .

Zhang, Y., Proenca, R., Maffei, M., Barone, M., Leopold, L. and Friedman, J. M. (1994). *Nature* **372**, 425–432.

3

The Mouse Genome

JEAN-LOUIS GUÉNET

*Institut Pasteur, 25 rue du Dr Roux, 75724 Paris,
Cedex 15, France*

Abstract

The mouse is an almost perfect model organism for the study of mammalian genomes. In addition to its ease of maintenance, short generation time and large litter size, several other characteristics are noteworthy.

(i) The ability to produce transgenic animals efficiently, either by injecting DNA sequences into one of the pronuclei of fertilized oocytes or by infecting embryonic stem (ES) cells *in vitro*.
(ii) The ability to alter the gene structure in the germline, either by injecting chemical mutagens or via homologous recombination in ES cells.
(iii) The possibility of producing various viable and fertile interspecific hybrids which allows the segregation of considerable genetic polymorphism in the progeny.

Several hundred mutants, exhibiting obesity with or without diabetes, hair loss or changed structure, dwarfism, skeletal defects, eye defects, inner ear defects, anaemia, metabolic diseases, neuromuscular or immunological disorders with more or less severe phenotypes, have been reported and many of these have proved interesting in the understanding of the developmental processes operating in mammals. A few of them, about 50, have been classified as 'homologous models', which means that homologies with human disease extend to the molecular level.

Within the last few years new methods in mapping of the mouse genome, which exploit the differences between genetically diverse *Mus* species and standard inbred strains, and which are based on the analysis of length polymorphism of polymerase chain reaction (PCR)-amplified sequences, have made possible the development of high resolution multilocus genetic linkage maps of the entire genome. Such maps, with an average of 200–400 molecular markers per chromosome, will allow the complete identification of regions of synteny between mouse and humans. They will

GENOMES, MOLECULAR BIOLOGY AND DRUG DISCOVERY
ISBN 0-12-137790-3

serve as an important tool for the rapid and efficient molecular analysis of mutant loci and they will also serve as the base for genome-wide physical mapping by allowing the ordering of overlapping sets (contigs) of large-sized DNA segments cloned in phages, cosmids or yeast artificial chromosomes (YACs).

In fact, the mouse will shortly become an organism where it will be possible and relatively easy to clone, by a positional approach, genes which have been identified by at least one mutant allele, and the only organism where it will be possible to test experimentally the biological role of virtually any sequences of unknown function.

In this respect it is not unrealistic to believe that the mouse may become the 'source of genes' for mammalian geneticists, just as *Arabidopsis thaliana* is for plant genetics.

1 Introduction

There is agreement among geneticists that the mouse is an almost perfect model organism because, in addition to its short generation time, ease of maintenance and high reproductive performance, it has several characteristics which, when considered together, make it unique. Among these characteristics three are particularly noteworthy in the context of this review.

First, the mouse is unusual in that it is possible to obtain strains which are homozygous at virtually all loci by repeatedly mating brothers to their sisters. Many such inbred strains have been established over the last decades. They have the advantage of producing only one type of gamete.

Second, the mouse is also unusual in that it is possible to produce viable and fertile hybrids by mating the above-mentioned highly inbred laboratory strains to various murine species derived from the wild. Crosses of this kind, as we shall see, have been extensively used for the establishment of the linkage map because they allow the segregation of a very large amount of genetic polymorphisms in a single cross.

Finally, an extensive knowledge of the early stages of mouse embryology has allowed the development of techniques for producing heritable alterations of the genome almost upon request. In the mouse it is relatively easy to produce efficiently transgenic animals by injecting DNA sequences (up to a few hundred kilobases in length) into one of the pronuclei of fertilized oocytes. It is also possible to substitute, in the germline, a 'mutant' copy of a given gene in place of the normal one via homologous recombination in embryonic stem (ES) cells. Transgenesis and homologous recombination have considerably strengthened the important role of the mouse as a model organism because they make it the only mammal in which one can test experimentally the biological role of DNA sequences of unknown function.

Being a model of choice the mouse has been extensively used by geneticists since the first experiments by Cuénot, who was first to report, in 1902, that Mendel's laws also applied to this species. Hundreds of mutations have been discovered and then assigned to a particular chromosome: this has resulted rapidly in a relatively dense linkage map. In the mid-1970s the discovery of new staining techniques for chromosomes allowed the allocation of each linkage group to a specific chromosome and its orientation with respect to the centromeric end. In 1980 the mouse had by far the most extensively documented genetic map of all mammalian species, including humans. With the advent of recombinant DNA technology and the development of entirely different approaches, the mouse lost its lead over human genetics but, at the same time, it has become clear that these two species were complementary from many points of view, and several large-scale programmes have been undertaken worldwide to support the rapid development of the mouse genetic maps. The aim of this review is to explain how these maps are established and what use they can be for human geneticists.

2 The mouse genome

The standard laboratory mouse has 40 chromosomes in its karyotype: 19 pairs of autosomes plus the two sex chromosomes. Mouse chromosomes are difficult to differentiate because, unlike human chromosomes, they are all acrocentric and exhibit a continuous gradation in size. In the laboratory a large number of chromosomal variants (inversions, deletions, reciprocal translocations etc.) have been induced, mostly by the use of chemical mutagens or as a consequence of irradiation. Others (Robertsonian translocations) have also been discovered in wild populations of Western Europe. A complete description of these chromosomal variants is provided in the book entitled *Genetic Variants and Strains of the Laboratory Mouse* (Lyon and Searle, 1989). We will not comment further on the use of these chromosomal variants but it is important to know that they played an important role in the late 1970s for the assignment of a particular linkage group to a specific mouse chromosome. They have also allowed the production of many types of trisomic genotypes and more recently they have contributed greatly to the discovery of the imprinting phenomenon.

The DNA content of the mouse haploid genome is 3 pg (3×10^{-12} g), which translates to 2.7×10^9 base pairs. If we consider that the genetic message is essentially composed of a succession of four nucleotides, symbolized A, G, C and T, with each of these nucleotides being equivalent to two bits of binary code information, one can easily calculate that the complete sequence of the mouse genome could be stored in the hard disk of a domestic PC.

Inside the mouse genome the 'genetic information', i.e. the fraction of DNA which is translated into proteins and regulatory sequences, is diluted in an ocean of DNA which has no known function. According to the most recent estimates no more than 5–8% of the DNA content is functional while the rest is represented by 'low complexity' sequences (the so-called satellite DNA) and a variety of repeated sequences of various sizes. Some of these sequences, particularly those which are short, have been very helpful for the establishment of the genetic maps, as we shall discuss later.

According to the most recent estimates the mouse genome contains between 50 000 and 120 000 genes, and probably no more than a few per cent of these genes have been identified either by a mutation or by molecular approaches (DNA sequencing). It is interesting to note, for example, that most of the new mutations which are discovered by 'mouse breeders' in general identify a new locus rather than a new allele at an already known locus. In this context, if we consider the recent data resulting from gene 'knock-out' experiments, it is likely that the majority of the mutations that occur in the mouse genome are either not detectable, because they are incompatible with a normal development of the embryo, or will not be detected because they have no obvious effect. This supports the contention that most of the genes packed into the mouse genome are still to be discovered, and it is likely that the development of high resolution/high density genetic maps of the genome will be very helpful.

3 Mapping the mouse genome

From a physical (and highly reductionist!) point of view genes are no more than little stretches of DNA which are lined along the chromosomes like the beads of a necklace. If we could label each of those 'molecular beads' specifically and then scan each chromosome from one end to the other at very high resolution with a very powerful apparatus, we could immediately assign to each gene a precise location on the chromosomes of a given species and accordingly establish at once an ultimate genetic map of the species. Establishing this sort of map, unfortunately, is not realistic with the techniques available at the present time. We know that there are thousands of genes tightly packed in the genome but, as already mentioned, very few of them are known in molecular terms. There is no way to label each of them specifically. We know that some genes are very large, with an irregular alternation of coding sequences (exons) and non-coding sequences (introns), while others are small. Finally we know that mammalian genomes are not as compact as most of the prokaryotic genomes, but are littered with repeated sequences of various kinds such as pseudogenes, proviral copies, minisatellites etc., the role of which (if any) is not clear. The high resolution 'chromosome scanner' that we would need for establishing our ultimate genetic map would then be extremely difficult to design.

Another way of establishing such an ultimate genetic map would be to clone the genome in small fragments, then carry out systematic sequencing of these fragments one after the other. This would eventually establish, in theory, the complete genome sequence of the species. Unfortunately this approach is not realistic either for a number of reasons. From previous experience we know, for example, that some parts of the genome would certainly be lost during the cloning step. We also know that this experiment would be a very tedious enterprise and probably also an enormous waste of money given that most of the sequenced material will be 'junk' or irrelevant.

The most reasonable way to develop a genetic map of the mouse genome is to develop it gradually, step by step, first by positioning a set of anchor loci (or markers), then by progressively increasing the number of markers in the intervals until we get a solid scaffold. With such a multistep approach, and provided that the number of markers available is large enough, it is possible to establish high resolution/high density maps of the genome. In fact, this is precisely the strategy that mouse geneticists have used since the beginning of the twentieth century, when J. B. S. Haldane and co-workers reported in the *Journal of Genetics* that two coat colour mutations, albino (*c*) and pink-eyed dilution (*p*) were linked (Haldane *et al.*, 1915).

3.1 The different maps of the mouse genome

There are three kinds of map which are of interest for geneticists: linkage maps, chromosome maps and physical maps.

3.1.1 Linkage maps

The establishment of a linkage map is based on the fact that, during meiosis, loci which are on different chromosomes assort randomly in the gametes while those which are on the same chromosome tend to co-segregate unless a cross-over splits the parental association. The probability for two genes to be separated by a cross-over event depends upon the genetic distance between them and this is reflected in the choice of the map unit, the centiMorgan (cM), which corresponds to a 1% chance of producing a recombinant gamete after one meiosis. A linkage map, in other words, is a diagrammatic representation of the linear arrangement of the genes which are located on a given chromosome.

Several points must be kept in mind concerning linkage maps.

 (i) Ordering loci on a linkage map requires, by definition, that at least one recombination event splits the parental linear arrangements. This is sometimes difficult to achieve if the two markers are tightly linked.
 (ii) The density of a linkage map is correlated to the number of polymorphisms which are segregated in a particular cross while its resolution depends upon the number of gametes (= total number of crossing over events) scored in the progeny.
(iii) The total length of the mouse linkage map has been estimated by several investigators, using different approaches, to be in the range 1550–1600 cM. This means that, on the average, 1 cM of the mouse genome corresponds to 1700 kb while in humans 1 cM roughly equals 1000 kb. These data must strictly be considered an average because there is no absolute correlation between cM and kb 'scales', because of the uneven distribution of the cross-overs along the chromatids. Two genes may appear completely linked on a high resolution map and turn out to be relatively distant from one another in molecular terms while, on the contrary, two genes may appear relatively distant from each other if there is a recombination 'hot spot' in the intergenic region.

3.1.2 Chromosomal maps

Whilst establishing linkage maps requires breeding experiments, chromosomal maps are established using techniques which do not require sexual reproduction.

These techniques are of three types: (i) *in situ* hybridization; (ii) somatic cell genetics; (iii) deletion mapping.

3.1.2.1 In situ hybridization. When a DNA sequence is labelled either with a fluorescent dye or with a radioactive isotope it is possible to hybridize it directly with the homologous sequence in the DNA of a specific chromosome and then to use the labelling to detect the sequence by direct observation of chromosome preparations under the microscope.

Even though *in situ* hybridization is a very reliable technique it has been much less used in the mouse than in humans essentially for three reasons: (i) in the mouse in most instances it is easier and faster to perform breeding experiments; (ii) it provides a regional assignment rather than a precise localization; (iii) mouse chromosomes, as mentioned above, are not easy to distinguish. *In situ* hybridization is however the technique of choice for the rapid localization of a transgene. It is also extremely useful to check if the large inserts of yeast artificial chromosomes (YACs) are all derived from the same chromosome or if they are chimeric.

3.1.2.2 Somatic cell genetics. Human–mouse somatic cell hybrids with a limited complement of human chromosomes, either intact or fragmented by heavy doses of irradiation, have been extensively used for chromosomal assignment of human genes. Similar hybrids segregating for the entire mouse chromosome also exist but have not been much used by mouse geneticists probably because, again, it is in general much easier and faster to rely on crosses, and also because, unlike in humans, somatic cell hybrids with deletions or translocations are rare, which complicates subchromosomal gene assignments by this approach.

3.1.2.3 Deletion mapping. Deletion mapping, whatever the species, is one of the most appealing ways to develop rapidly a very precise map for a small chromosomal region. However, the technique requires that a set of overlapping deletions of various sizes be available in the region in question, and that complementation tests be made in order to get an estimate of the size of these deletions. Such deletion maps have already been established in three regions of the mouse genome: albino (*c*; chromosome 7), dilute short-ear (*d-se*; chromosome 9) and in the *T/t* region of mouse chromosome 17. In all three instances they have provided a lot of information and have allowed the identification of many new genes (Moore *et al.*, 1988). Even though very powerful mutagens which produce deletions in the genome are available in the arsenal of mouse geneticists, this strategy is unfortunately limited in its application.

3.1.3 Physical maps
A physical map is an accurate representation of the linear arrangement of the genes on a chromosome. The gene order is the same as that given by the genetic map but the distance between genes is measured in kb or Mb. Physical maps represent a crucial step in the structural and functional characterization of the mouse genome. They can be achieved

by several methods but the most convenient consists of ordering overlapping sets (contigs) of large-sized DNA segments cloned in phages (λ or P1 in general), cosmids, bacterial artificial chromosomes (BACs) or yeast artificial chromosomes (YACs).

Although it is possible, at least in theory, to develop a physical map *de novo*, for example by cloning the ends of the mouse DNA insert of a particular YAC or P1 clone, then detecting other clones with these ends as a probe, then repeating the operation over and over until many cloned DNA segments can be ordered in a head-to-tail manner, the establishment of such a map is greatly facilitated when a high density linkage map with an average of 200–400 molecular markers per chromosome already exits. In this strategy the establishment of a physical map is a second step after the linkage map has been established.

As for linkage maps, several points must be kept in mind concerning physical maps.

(i) Before establishing YAC or P1 contigs it is important to confirm that each of the cloned DNA molecules really represents unaltered stretches of DNA deriving from one chromosome only. Given that all libraries are made with the same basic strategy (which uses first the action of a restriction endonuclease to fragment the high molecular weight DNA and then the ligation of the digestion products in a vector), it is quite common that, by chance, two completely independent segments are packed together, in a head-to-tail arrangement, in the same yeast cell. The resulting YAC is mosaic and its uncritical use may be misleading. A similar, although more perverse situation, can also occur when a piece of DNA is deleted in the YAC.

(ii) In order to establish contigs of overlapping YACs, BACs, cosmids or P1 clones it is necessary that several independent YAC libraries be constructed with various restriction enzymes and complete or incomplete digestions. In the mouse several such libraries exist representing at least 15 genome equivalents. In these conditions one expects that a given probe will match with 15 clones on average. Unfortunately this not the case and some segments of the mouse genome are not represented in the available libraries. It will therefore be very difficult to bring the physical map of the mouse genome to complete 'closure'.

3.2 Integrating the maps

From a given cross one can establish a linkage map only for the set of markers which segregate in it but, unfortunately, the number of such genetic markers is always limited. It is limited either by the polymorphisms which exist in the parents or by the technique(s) which is used for their detection, and it is therefore important to merge results from several independent crosses into the same consensus map. This is possible when the data collected from independent crosses have markers in common. To help in the integration of the different maps, mouse geneticists have defined a set of anchor loci which are evenly distributed over the different chromosomes and are highly polymorphic.

4 Markers used for the construction of genetic (linkage) maps

Any kind of change in the DNA sequence making an individual or group of individuals different from the other members of the same species can be considered a potential genetic marker, provided we have tools to recognize and follow it, either directly or indirectly, generation after generation. The genetic markers which have been used by mouse geneticists, even if they have changed since the early days, have always been selected on three major criteria: abundance, simplicity of typing and cost. We will describe here only a few of these markers, with emphasis on those which have proven the most helpful.

4.1 Markers scored by gross examination of the external phenotype

As mentioned earlier the mouse linkage map began to be established in 1915 with the observation by Haldane and co-workers that the albino locus (*c*) was linked to the pink eye dilution locus (*p*). Since this initial observation, the genetic map has progressively become more and more dense as a consequence of the continuous discovery of new mutant alleles at different loci scattered throughout the mouse genome. Accumulation of these new mutant alleles was, in part, a direct consequence of the use of the mouse as a model organism for the evaluation of the genetic effects of radiation or genotoxic chemicals, and in part also an indirect consequence of the choice of inbreeding as a mating system for the maintenance of most of the standardized strains of laboratory mice because inbreeding, although it has no effect on the mutation rate, makes the detection of spontaneously occurring recessive mutations more frequent.

Over 150 mutant alleles with an obvious effect on eye or coat colour, skeleton morphology, behaviour, fur texture, etc. have contributed to the establishment of the backbone of today's linkage map and some of them, as discussed later, are still very useful markers. Unfortunately these markers have two main drawbacks.

(i) They frequently impair the viability and/or the fertility of the affected animals and, for this reason, it is extremely difficult to set up crosses with more than three or four markers of this type segregating at one time.

(ii) Even if the great majority of the mutations which occur *de novo* in the mouse identify new loci instead of a new allele at already known loci, their total number remains relatively limited.

Mutant alleles which are recognizable by gross examination of the external phenotype are interesting because of their effects on development or as models of human genetic diseases, but they no longer represent an important source of genetic markers.

4.2 Proteins with similar functions but different primary structures

From the late 1960s onwards the development of gel electrophoresis and the concomitant discovery of techniques for staining the product(s) of enzymatic reactions allowed the identification of new loci attributable to polymorphisms resulting from discrete variations in the electric charge of proteins. This type of molecular marker, referred to as electromorphs or electrophoretic variants, has three advantages over the classical visible phenotype markers: (i) they are co-dominantly expressed and can then be typed in heterozygotes; (ii) they are in general compatible with a normal function of the enzyme and accordingly do not impair the viability or fertility of the animals; (iii) they are relatively abundant, probably as they are selectively neutral, and therefore allow a wide coverage of the genome.

There are now well over 100 markers of this kind which are amenable to laboratory analysis, and new variants are regularly discovered, particularly in wild mice. These markers have enabled the rapid development of the mouse linkage map but, unfortunately, they have the drawback that they require a relatively complex technique to characterize each of them and this makes large-scale linkage experiments based on this approach expensive to run. We must also remember that no more than 10% of the genomic DNA is actually translated into proteins, and no more than a few per cent of these proteins can mutate without impairing the viability of the carrier. It is thus obvious that even if the proteins were, directly or indirectly, the only possible polymorphic markers available for the purpose of gene mapping this would be insufficient for the development of high resolution maps.

4.3 Polymorphisms detected at the DNA level

The advent of recombinant DNA technology and the increasing number of studies carried out on the structure of genomic DNA have opened the way to the development of an entirely new type of genetic marker. Among these markers are those which are generated by the restriction endonucleases, e.g. restriction fragment length polymorphisms (RFLPs), and those which are detected by polymerase chain reaction (PCR) amplification of specific segments. We will consider each of these in turn.

4.3.1 Markers generated by restriction endonucleases

4.3.1.1 Restriction fragment length polymorphisms. Strategies used for the establishment of mammalian genetic maps changed dramatically in 1981 when Botstein and co-workers reported that the fragments generated by restriction endonuclease digestion of DNA samples of different individuals, when separated by gel electrophoresis and identified by hybridization with labelled molecular probes, often exhibited size polymorphisms. These polymorphisms, the RFLPs, like the electrophoretic variants described above, behave as co-dominant Mendelian characters and accordingly can be used for linkage analysis.

RFLPs exploit the variation in size of DNA fragments generated by the specific action of the restriction endonucleases which have the property of cutting the DNA in a non-random manner but, in contrast to other markers, RFLPs have the advantage of being extremely abundant since every event which alters a restriction site can potentially be detected. They also have the advantage of requiring only one technique for processing the same sample of high molecular weight DNA. From this point of view, Botstein's strategy must be considered a landmark breakthrough in gene mapping technology.

Over the last 10 years, RFLPs associated with various probes (cloned genes or anonymous sequences) have been extensively used as genetic markers and they are still used for the chromosomal assignment of recently cloned cDNAs.

At this point it is interesting to note that RFLP analysis requires neither the discovery of a mutant allele nor even the expression of a particular gene for its localization to be possible.

The probe/restriction fragment pair can be considered as a marker which is normally unique for the genome since the probability of finding two sequences giving a restriction fragment of the same size and having a similar affinity for a given probe is very small, at least in normal circumstances. An exception occurs if a molecular probe corresponds to a (coding or non-coding) sequence which is repeated several times in the mouse genome, when all the generated RFLPs will each identify only one apparent locus. This is the case, for example, for some pseudogenes, which are present as several copies inside the genome (Siracusa *et al.*, 1991), and also for some other repeated sequences (Stoye and Coffin, 1988; Taylor and Rowe, 1989; Hastie, 1989).

4.3.1.2 Restriction landmark genomic scanning. The restriction landmark genomic scanning (RLGS) technique (Hayashizaki *et al.*, 1994) is based on the use of radiolabelled specific restriction sites as markers. Although several variations have been reported the technique consists in general of six successive steps.

  (i) A sample of high molecular weight DNA is digested with an 8 bp or 10 bp cutter (in general *Not*I, which is an 8 bp cutter) in order to produce large-sized digestion products (average size of these fragments in mouse DNA is around 1 Mb).
 (ii) The digested fragments are end-labelled with radioactive dideoxynucleotide.
(iii) The fragments are digested a second time with a 6 bp cutter.
 (iv) The digestion products are resolved by electrophoresis in agarose.
  (v) The mixture of the digested products is digested a last time with a 4 bp cutter.
 (vi) Finally the short restriction fragments are resolved by polyacrylamide gel electrophoresis (PAGE). The number of restriction fragments increases by the successive actions of the second and third enzymes but only those which are end-labelled will be recognized on final autoradiography.

Although it requires very rigorous technical conditions RLGS is a very clever technique which may become very useful for high resolution mapping of specific regions.

4.3.2 Markers detectable by PCR
Since the observation by Botstein several other techniques have been reported

which are also based on the analysis of structural variations at the DNA level. Among the most interesting are those which take advantage of PCR, because they require very small quantities of template DNA and can be carried out within only a few hours. The most popular of these techniques consist of the amplification of short sequences (usually less than 300 bp) whose polymorphisms are either in length (simple sequence length polymorphisms (SSLPs) or microsatellites) or in the sequence itself (single strand conformation polymorphisms (SSCPs), denaturing gradient gel electrophoresis (DGGE).

4.3.2.1 Simple sequence length polymorphisms. SSLPs or 'microsatellites' are composed of short tandem repeats of 1–4 base long units, such as $(T)_n$, $(CA)_n$, $(CT)_n$, $(CAG)_n$, etc. Their origin is on the whole unknown but it makes sense to suppose that they may result either from errors occurring during DNA replication, a sort of 'stuttering of the DNA polymerase', or from unequal recombinational events. The size polymorphisms can be assessed by agarose gel electrophoresis or PAGE after PCR amplification using specific primers designed from the sequences flanking the repeats (Love *et al.,* 1990; Hearne *et al.,* 1991; Montagutelli *et al.,* 1991).

These microsatellites represent almost ideal molecular markers because: (i) they are usually found in the non-coding regions and the polymorphisms therefore are less likely to alter phenotype; (ii) they are numerous (probably about 10^5 copies for CA repeats); (iii) they are evenly distributed throughout the genome; (iv) they are relatively stable generation after generation.

Thanks to the efforts of the team lead by Dr Eric Lander (Dietrich *et al.,* 1992, 1994) at the Whitehead Institute in Boston, mouse geneticists now have access to a collection of over 6000 such microsatellite markers. This is more than sufficient to develop a high density molecular linkage map of the mouse genome. These markers are universal and their sequence has been published. They can be used both for the identification of polymorphic loci on the mouse linkage map and for the identification of a YAC or P1 clone in a library.

4.3.2.2 Single strand conformation polymorphisms and denaturing gradient gel electrophoresis. Structural polymorphisms of PCR products can also be assayed by comparing the electrophoretic mobility in a polyacrylamide gel after denaturation (SSCP) or by measuring their migration within a polyacrylamide gel containing a gradient of denaturing compounds such as urea and formamide (DGGE). In these two cases the method is so sensitive that a change of only a single base pair in the sequence of an 80–250 bp long DNA molecule is detectable.

4.3.2.3 Other markers detectable by PCR assay. Many other strategies have been used in the mouse to identify polymorphic loci. Most of them have no real advantage over the microsatellites, which have now become universal, and we will only report here the use of the so-called random amplified polymorphic DNAs (RAPDs) because this type of marker may become useful for the establishment of physical maps. The technique for RAPDs is based on the use of single, arbitrarily designed short oligomers as PCR primers with a modified amplification protocol. Following pilot experiments carried out first by Williams *et al.* (1990) and then by Welsh *et al.* (1991) we and others found that, when such short oligonucleotides (10-mers), of 50–70% G + C content, were used for PCR amplification of genomic DNA templates of various origins, half of these primers generated strain-specific polymorphic products (ranging from 0.3 to 0.6 kb) which could easily be localized on the mouse genome (Serikawa *et al.*, 1992). Used in pairs these primers also generated additional polymorphic products which could also be mapped.

Despite the lack of information on the sequence or locus analysed, and the fact that a given product may be observed in one strain or species without any equivalent being detected in another, this technique offers the major advantage of providing geneticists with an almost unlimited number of markers at very low cost. Since it does not require preliminary data about genes or sequences it should be especially useful for species where the genetic map and the availability of sequence data are still very poor.

To summarize this section, a tremendous range of 'cryptic' polymorphisms are available, and techniques to identify them are numerous and relatively easy to use. Geneticists thus have in hand all the tools necessary to undertake the establishment of high density linkage maps. To make these maps high resolution maps depends significantly upon the number of meioses studied and upon the strategy used.

5   Strategies for the establishment of genetic (linkage) maps

Mouse geneticists use the same strategies as human geneticists for the establishment of chromosomal and physical maps. For the establishment of linkage maps, however, they use specific strategies which we will briefly report here. All these strategies are the direct consequence of the fact that in the mouse: (i) it is possible to set up crosses at will; (ii) it is possible to use inbred lines which produce only one type of gamete; (iii) it is possible to breed an unlimited number of offspring from a certain type of cross.

However one point must be kept in mind: in the mouse, as in humans, the indispensable element of a linkage study is heterozygosity. Only if an individual is heterozygous at each of two loci can the linkage relationship between these two loci be established.

5.1   Backcrosses and intercrosses

Even if 'non-sexual' techniques have occasionally been used in mouse genetics, most of the data which have contributed to the establishment of the genetic maps of the species result from informative crosses. These crosses are of two types: backcrosses and intercrosses.

Backcrosses are very easy to analyse because, by definition, each animal of a progeny produces a single gamete. If A and B are two markers which are being tested for linkage, with two alleles at the A locus (a and a') and two alleles at the B locus (b and b') the backcross $a/a'-b/b' \times a/a-b/b$ will produce four genotypes: $a/a'-b/b'$; $a/a-b/b$; $a/a'-b/b$; and $a/a-b/b'$; in equal proportions if the markers are unlinked. If, on the contrary, the two markers are linked (symbolized: $ab/a'b' \times ab/ab$) the backcross will produce a proportion of offspring with recombinant genotypes which will be the direct consequence of the linkage tightness. If f is the observed number of recombinant genotypes among the offspring and n the total number of animals in the sample, the value of r (the percentage of recombination) is given by the formula:

$$r = \frac{f}{n}$$

The standard error of r is given by the formula:

$$SE_r = \sqrt{\frac{r(1-r)}{n}}$$

With such a formula one can compute that a backcross panel of 300 progeny provides a 95% probability of recombining genes that are 1.0 cM apart and a 460 progeny panel provides a 99% probability of recombination in that distance. One can also conclude that two genes exhibiting complete linkage in a progeny of 1000 offspring are at a distance of less than 0.3 cM at the 5% risk level. This would mean that they have a great probability of being cloned within the same YAC.

Intercrosses are much less used in mouse genetics than backcrosses. They do however have the advantage that every offspring results from two gametes instead of one.

5.2 Recombinant inbred strains

Recombinant inbred strains (RISs) (Taylor, 1978) are produced by systematic and unrelaxed inbreeding of the successive offspring of any two individuals of an interstrain F2, mated at random. When these animals are to be used for the purpose of gene mapping some points must be kept in mind.

(i) Being inbred, each strain of an RIS set represents a collection of individuals with identical genomes, homozygous for all of their genes, which can be bred in unlimited numbers. They also remain stable generation after generation with the only exception of possible new mutations.

(ii) Having origins in two unrelated progenitor strains they have, by definition, inherited every component of their genetic make-up either from one or the other strain. In other words, at the genetic level, each line looks like a patchwork made up of chromosomal fragments derived, at random, from the two progenitor strains. Those genes which are linked on the same chromosome have a tendency to remain associated through successive generations except when a cross-over splits the association.

When an RIS is being established, crossing-over events can occur at every generation, in each sexual partner, as long as a chromosomal segment of a given parental origin is variable in size among the different individuals of a given strain. The chromosomes are thus progressively chopped into small-sized segments, much smaller than those resulting from a single meiotic process although, on average, any individual RIS is homozygous for 50% of the alleles coming from a progenitor strain just like any backcross progeny.

RISs are very useful for the detection of linkage because all the data collected may be used additively. The results collected with markers A and B for example can be used for the mapping of markers C, D, etc.

Several sets of recombinant inbred strains are available for mapping experiments and a complete list of these strains appears in Lyon and Searle (1989). The most used are BXD (inbred parents C57BL/6J and DBA/2J), AXB–BXA (inbred parents C57BL/6J and A/J), and AKXL (inbred parents AKR/J and C57BL/6J).

When a new marker gene is to be typed using the RIS strategy, polymorphism is first checked for among the parental strains, then when a suitable difference is observed each strain of the set is typed. The strain distribution pattern (SDP) for the new polymorphism is matched to the former SDPs stored in the databases, then both the position of the new marker and its linkage with the flanking markers is calculated.

The recombinant frequency r is given by the formula:

$$r = \frac{R}{(4-6R)}$$

where R is the ratio of 'recombinant' strains, for a pair of adjacent genes, relative to the total number of RISs.

RIS is an ideal tool for the detection of relatively tight linkages (no 'recombinant' genotype for example); while on the other hand, cross–intercross or cross–backcross protocols are more appropriate to detect linkages over distances greater than 10 cM.

6 Wild mice as a source of polymorphisms

With the increasing use of molecular markers for the development of the mouse linkage map, it rapidly became clear that the common laboratory mouse strains were not as polymorphic as were other mammalian species, such as humans. RFLPs, for example, appeared to be much less common in the genome of the classical inbred mouse strains than in the human genome where some estimates have put the frequency as high as 1 in 100 bp. In the same way only 50% of the microsatellite markers cloned from the mouse genome are polymorphic among laboratory strains, while in humans, this percentage is close to 90%. These observations in fact were consistent with many historical records indicating that most of the inbred laboratory strains were derived from a very limited number of progenitors (Bonhomme *et al.,* 1987). To bypass this relative deficiency in polymorphisms mouse geneticists thought, about 10 years ago, that it might be interesting to use wild specimens of the same genus *Mus* to cross with the laboratory strains. This idea, as we shall see, has opened a new era in mouse genetics: the 'interspecific backcross' era.

The first wild specimens used for the purpose of gene mapping were from the *Mus spretus* species. *Mus spretus* is a wild species of mouse which is quite common on the western part of the Mediterranean border (Bonhomme and Guénet, 1989) and whose habitat is completely different from that of *Mus musculus domesticus*. It is the most distantly related species of the genus *Mus* that still interbreeds with laboratory strains (Fig. 1) to produce fertile hybrids (Bonhomme *et al.,* 1978), and crosses of this species with laboratory inbred strains have become a method of choice for generating multilocus linkage maps. In general the production of interspecific hybrids results from natural matings between laboratory strain females and *Mus spretus* males, although some hybrids have also been produced with the opposite cross-configuration either by artificial insemination or by *in vitro* fertilization. F1 males are sterile, as a consequence of the Haldane effect, but F1 females are fertile

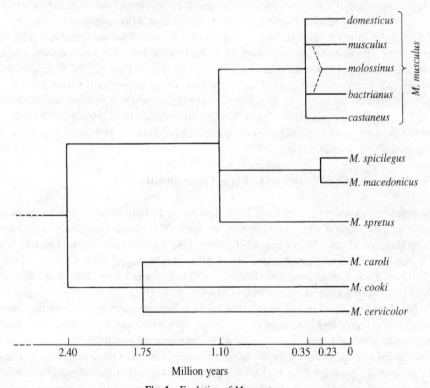

Fig. 1 Evolution of *Mus* genus.

and can be used to produce a backcross generation by mating them to males of either the laboratory strain or of the wild species.

The mapping strategy using *Mus spretus* hybrids is reliable and has been proved by several investigators not to introduce any widespread bias into gene localization. It can be applied in all circumstances where a probe is available since the discovery of a suitable restriction polymorphism is generally not a problem. In a study carried out in our laboratory we found for example that the four enzymes *Bgl*II, *Msp*I, *Taq*I and *Xba*I allowed the identification of easy-to-score RFLPs with 81% of a set of randomly cloned DNA sequences. With PCR-based techniques it should be noticed however that, as a consequence of the evolutionary divergence, some oligonucleotides designed from a sequence established from a laboratory strain may fail to prime (or may not prime using the same conditions) amplification of the homologous *Mus spretus* DNA segment.

With more refined techniques, such as those based on the analysis of discrete structural variation, which are capable of detecting a single base replacement (SSCP and DGGE), it is likely that virtually any DNA stretch from a non-coding region of more than 100 bp long will be found to be polymorphic between *Mus spretus* and any other strain.

With the increasing emphasis of techniques based on PCR amplification for the detection of genetic polymorphism, several other species of the *Mus* genus which are less distantly related to the laboratory strains than *Mus spretus* have also been found to be of great value. Using a large set of microsatellites we found that 82% of the latter allowed the amplification of polymorphic products between the PWK inbred strain, derived from *Mus musculus musculus*, and the C57BL/6 laboratory strain. More interestingly, we found that this strain appeared (by this criterion) almost as distantly related to *Mus spretus* as to the common laboratory strains (82% vs 70%) (Montagutelli *et al.*, 1991). Similar observation have been made by others using the substrains *Mus musculus castaneus* (Dietrich *et al.*, 1994) and *Mus musculus molossinus* (Harada *et al.*, 1989).

7 Analysing the results of linkage experiments

Several computer programs have been developed to help mouse geneticists store and analyse data from experimental crosses. The most commonly used are MapMaker/EXP and MapMaker/QTL, from Eric Lander (Whitehead Institute for Biomedical Research, Cambridge, MA, USA), MapManager, from Kenneth Manly (Roswell Park Cancer Institute, Buffalo, NY, USA) and Gene-Link, from Xavier Montagutelli (Institut Pasteur, Paris, France).

MapMaker/EXP (Lincoln *et al.*, 1992a) is a linkage analysis package for constructing primary linkage maps of dominant, recessive, and co-dominant markers segregating in BC1 backcrosses, F2 and F3 intercrosses and RISs. It performs full multipoint linkage analyses, i.e. a simultaneous estimation of all recombination fractions from the primary data. It also incorporates an algorithm for detecting potential genotyping errors (Lincoln and Lander, 1992) and has the ability to draw maps as

PostScript graphics. MapMaker/QTL (Lincoln *et al.*, 1992b) is a companion program to MapMaker/EXP which allows the mapping of genes controlling polygenic quantitative traits in F2 intercrosses and BC1 backcrosses relative to a genetic linkage map. Both programs can be run on Sun SPARC Stations, IBM PC compatibles or Apple Macintosh with A/UX. They can be obtained free of charge from the ftp site: genome.wi.mit.edu or from the Web site: http://www-genome.wi.mit.edu.

MapManager (Manly, 1993) is a Macintosh program providing functions to collect and analyse data from BC1 backcrosses, F2 intercrosses and RISs. It has several database functions that help in organizing and manipulating data conveniently. It is able to build maps using a simulated annealing procedure. Recently, a set of functions has been added to analyse quantitative traits by analysis of variance. MapManager can be obtained from the author (e-mail: kmanly@mcbio.med.buffalo.edu) under license.

Gene-Link (Montagutelli, 1990) is a linkage program to analyse data from BC1 backcrosses. It performs multipoint linkage analyses (up to six loci) and can look for transmission ratio distortion and epistatic relationships. A new version released in 1995 has several functions to manage complex mapping projects. It can be obtained free of charge from the author by e-mail (xmonta@pasteur.fr).

These different programs can only deal with one type of cross at a time. When one wishes to combine genetic data from a backcross and an intercross, it is necessary to use human genetic linkage programs such as LINKAGE (Lathrop and Lalouel, 1984; Terwilliger and Ott, 1992), CRIMAP (Lander and Green, 1987) or its automated enhancement MULTIMAP (Matise *et al.*, 1994). For a review of these programs and their availability, readers are referred to the *Guide to Human Genome Computing* (Bishop, 1994). Data obtained from RISs and any other cross have to be analysed separately and results combined by hand.

8 The large-scale mapping programmes

Several large-scale mapping programmes have been developed over the last 10 years. Details of the most important are given.

Historically, two projects have been developed for the mapping of molecular markers on the mouse genome. Both were based on interspecific backcrosses involving the *Mus spretus* species and the laboratory strain C57BL/6. The first project was set up at the Institut Pasteur (Guénet *et al.*, 1988), the other at the Frederick Cancer Research and Development Center (Copeland and Jenkins, 1991; Copeland *et al.*, 1993).

Since then, two other programmes have been developed, one at the Jackson Laboratory and a second one on the basis of a cooperation between the British MRC and the Institut Pasteur in Paris (the European Collaborative Interspecific Backcross or EUCIB; Breen *et al.*, 1994). The DNA panel at the Jackson Laboratory consists of two sets of 96 samples prepared from two reciprocal interspecific crosses involving *Mus spretus*. The EUCIB resource is by far the largest panel in the world, consisting of 982 samples that have been typed for anchor markers across the entire mouse genome. This programme provides a unique resource for the high resolution genetic mapping, and subsequent physical mapping, of the mouse and human genomes (Breen *et al.,* 1994). Both panels (the one from the Jackson Laboratory and the one of the EUCIB consortium) are available for the purpose of mapping.

9 Applications of the mouse genetic maps

Genetic maps have in common with the systematics of living organisms that their usefulness is not obvious to the untutored mind. In this section we will highlight, with the help of a few selected examples, some of the most important applications of the maps for current and future genome research.

9.1 The use of the linkage map for the identification of specific genotypes

Breeding mouse mutants for the purpose of research is often made difficult by the fact that homozygous genotypes, which are particularly useful for research, are either sterile or severely affected and accordingly unable to breed. This is the case, for example, for the vast majority of neurological or muscular mutations which, in general, are incompatible with more than a few days of life *ab utero.* This is also the case for the mutation inducing obesity where the affected mice cannot breed. Here the genetic map, as we shall see, can be very helpful. Let us consider, for example, the mouse mutation progressive motor neuronopathy (*pmn*) which is an autosomal recessive mutation characterized by a progressive neurogenic muscular atrophy of the caudo-cranial type. Homozygotes can be identified between day 14 and day 20 after birth, when they begin to develop paralysis of the hind limbs; between day 35 and day 42 they become completely paralysed and finally die between day 50 and day 55 (Schmalbruch *et al.,* 1991). The pathology of this mutation is reminiscent of the picture observed in the Werdnig–Hoffmann type of infantile spinal muscular atrophy in humans, and mainly for this reason the *pmn* mutation has been considered an excellent animal model. Mapping experiments have localized *pmn* very close ($\leq$0.2 cM) to the extra toe locus (*Xt*) on mouse chromosome 13 (Bueno Brunialti *et al.,* 1995). This localization has permitted an increase in the efficiency of the breeding stocks by allowing the establishment of balanced stocks of the type *Xt* +/+ *pmn*. Given that recombination between the two loci *Xt* and *pmn* occurs at very low frequency, crosses of that kind produce three genotypes: one-fourth of the conceptuses (those which are *Xt* +/*Xt* +) die *in utero*, one-fourth (those which are homozygous for the mutant allele of interest, + *pmn*/+ *pmn*) develop the neurological syndrome from the age of 2 weeks onwards and the remaining half of the conceptuses are heterozygous carriers (*Xt* +/+ *pmn*) like their parents, and are easily scorable by analysing their hind limbs where an extra digit is clearly visible. Such an intercross, which allows the identification of the homozygous + *pmn*/+ *pmn* progeny well before the onset of the degenerating process, is of paramount importance for neurobiologists wishing to study the evolution in the pathology of the degenerative progress. It is also important for researchers who are experimenting with gene therapies of various kinds (Sendtner *et al.*, 1992).

9.2 Evolution at the genome level

Inside the mouse genome, as discussed at the beginning of this chapter, several sequences appear to be repeated a number of times. Some of these sequences are functional genes and, when the different copies of these genes are localized on chromosomes, two situations may be observed: either they are on the same chromosome at a relatively short distance or they map to different chromosomes. Such distribution clearly results from evolutionary changes which have occurred at the genome level at various times in the history of the species. They are not completely understood yet but, with the rapid development of genetic maps, we should be able to understand better what happened during evolution.

Genes which are repeated in tandem on the same chromosome very likely result from duplications of an ancestral gene. In the mouse genome there are numerous examples where one copy of the duplicated gene is active in one tissue while the other copy is active in another tissue. This is the case for the genes encoding amylases (*Amy1* and *Amy2*) which map to chromosome 3. These two genes clearly result from the duplication of a common ancestor, but one is active in the salivary glands (*Amy1*) while the other is active in pancreas (*Amy2*). Other situations are even more interesting, for example the renin genes *Ren1* and *Ren2*, on mouse chromosome 1, where some mouse strains have only one copy of the gene while others have two. In this case the gene duplication seems to be a recent event because it is not yet fixed in the *Mus musculus domesticus* species itself.

Gene duplications sometimes result from chromosomal segment duplication followed by translocation. This is the case, for example, for two pieces of mouse chromosome, one from chromosome 11 and the other from chromosome 15, which both exhibit the same linear arrangement for three related genes: *Rara*, *Hox2* and *Krt1* on chromosome 11; *Rarg*, *Hox3* and *Krt2* on chromosome 15. In this case, which is termed a paralogy, the two chromosomal segments obviously had a common ancestor because it is very unlikely that such a linear arrangement could have occurred by chance. A similar situation also exists in the human genome where the homologous genes are located respectively on chromosome 17q and 12q with the same linear arrangement as the mouse.

As more and more multigene families are identified and mapped on the mouse genetic map, as well as in other mammalian species, the evolutionary mechanisms involved in genome modelling will be easier to understand.

9.3 Interspecific chromosomal homologies

Around 3000 gene loci are now mapped in the mouse (*Mammalian Genome*, 1994), and a similar number in humans. Of these, about 1000 homologous genes are mapped or assigned to chromosomes in both species (Nadeau *et al.*, 1992;

Mammalian Genome, 1994), and it can be seen that there are groups of genes which exhibit the same linear ordering in the two species. Each of these groups constitutes a conserved autosomal segment or interspecific chromosomal homology. At present there are over 110 such segments which range in genetic length from less than 1 cM to over 50 cM. The total length of all conserved autosomal segments is about 980 cM which corresponds to about 61% of the mouse genome. On different human chromosomes the number of conserved segments ranges from one to seven and on mouse chromosomes from 3 to 12.

Such comparative maps can be used to predict linkages and identify candidate disease genes both in humans and in the mouse. A recent example of this was reported in a 1994 issue of *Genomics* (Montagutelli *et al.,* 1994; Janocha *et al.,* 1994) where the mapping of the mouse homologue of the metabolic disease alkaptonuria (the *aku* mutation) on mouse chromosome 16 helped in the localization of the human defect on human chromosome 3. Another example where the mapping of a gene in the mouse has helped in the identification of the underlying gene for a human mutation is the mapping of *Pax3* to chromosome 1 in the mouse, in a conserved linkage group that contains the gene for Waardenburg syndrome type 1 (Sicinski *et al.,* 1989). Identification of peripherin as the gene underlying the *rds* (retinal degeneration slow) mutation in the mouse also suggested the homologous human RDS gene as a strong candidate for one form of autosomal dominant retinitis pigmentosa in the human population.

A good knowledge of the gene order inside the homologous segments in two different species can also be used to transfer linkage information from species such as humans and mice to other species such as cattle, pig, sheep etc.

9.4 Analysis of complex traits

The determinism of many diseases of humans, such as infectious diseases, autoimmune diseases, diabetes, susceptibility to drug addiction etc., is often controlled by more than one gene, and it is obvious that the identification of these genes and determination of their function could open entirely new opportunities for medical intervention. In fact the identification of these genes is often easier in mice than in humans. Once a candidate disease gene or disease region is identified in the mouse, the homologous genes or regions in humans can be screened to see if they are linked to the corresponding human genetic disease.

9.5 Positional cloning of classical mouse mutations

Cloning of a gene which is known by its phenotype but not by the protein it codes for (a strategy which is often called 'positional cloning' or 'reverse genetics', probably because its proceeds from the phenotype to the gene) implies that the gene in question be isolated in a vector with the smallest possible amount of irrelevant flanking DNA. This requires, first, the establishment of a high density map in the upstream and downstream regions of the gene together with the identification of the two closest markers to avoid unnecessary work in the final steps of the identification of the gene. Many genes exist in the mouse which are very interesting either because they are models of human genetic diseases or simply because they alter an essential function in mammalian development: many of them are now in the process of being cloned by a positional approach. A good example is provided by the recent cloning of the obese gene which has been achieved by scientists in Friedman's laboratory in New York (Zhang *et al.*, 1994). Obese (*ob*) maps to mouse chromosome 6 and is characterized by an enormous enlargement of body weight in affected homozygotes due to an increased intake of food. Researchers in Friedman's team first developed a very precise map of the region and then, with the help of this map, identified several YACs and P1 clones overlapping the *ob* gene and finally identified a new gene, the product of which is involved in the genetic control of satiety and energy expenditure.

Other mutations are sometimes identified in molecular terms by the so-called candidate gene approach, which works as follows. A gene, which is known in the form of a mutant allele, is placed on the mouse map while concurrently a cDNA is also mapped in the region and a plausible connection is first suspected and then examined. The first example of this case was provided by scientists in Gruss' laboratory, in Göttingen (Chalepakis *et al.*, 1991), who reported that the homeobox containing the gene *Pax1*, which was found to map to chromosome 2 in a region where the old mutation undulated (*un*) had been mapped a long time before, was indeed the target of the mutation in the affected animals. A more recent example (Gibson *et al.*, 1995) is the mouse mutation shaker-1 (*sha1*) which was found to be the consequence of a mutation in a gene encoding a new type of myosin. This result was confirmed by human geneticists who demonstrated that the homologous gene of humans was responsible for Usher syndrome type 1B (Weil *et al.*, 1995).

With the rapid increase in marker density on mouse genetic maps and the availability of several large-insert YAC libraries, it is now possible to undertake the positional cloning of virtually any mutation. This requires however that the mutation of interest first be precisely positioned with respect to several flanking markers.

9.6 Validation of mouse models for human genetic diseases

The discovery of mouse mutations with a pathology reminiscent of that associated with a human syndrome is a relatively common situation. In the mouse, for example, there are at least 10 mutations inducing motor neuron degeneration which have been reported (Bronson *et al.*, 1992): wobbler (*wr*, chromosome 11), motor neuron degeneration (*mnd*, chromosome 8), motor neuron degeneration-2 (*mnd2*, chromosome 6), muscle deficient (*mdf*, chromosome 19), neuromuscular degeneration (*nmd*, chromosome 19), lumbosacral neuroaxonal dystrophy (*lnd*, chromosome 7), gracile axonal dystrophy (*gad*, chromosome 5), wasted (*wst*, chromosome 2), generalized neuroaxonal dystrophy (*gnd*) and progressive motor neuronopathy (*pmn*) (Schmalbruch *et al.*, 1991). Most of these mutations have been studied in detail and all of them exhibit a rather specific phenotype at the histological level. They also exhibit a great range in severity indicating that, in each case, neuronal degeneration probably results from a specific process. However none of these mutations maps to a mouse chromosomal region known to be syntenic with a region where a human disease has been localized. The consequence of this is that, with the exception of *mnd*, which is recognized as a model of neuronal ceroid lipofuscinosis or Batten disease (Bronson *et al.*, 1993), no truly homologous model is available for any of the human motor neuronopathies. This also indicates that neuronal integrity must depend on the functioning of a great number of mammalian genes, and in this respect all the mouse mutations which have been accumulated over time represent potentially invaluable tools. A similar situation also exists with Hirschsprung disease, where at least three analogous mouse models are known (lethal spotting (*ls*, chromosome 2), piebald lethal (*s^l*, chromosome 14) and dominant megacolon (*Dom*, chromosome 15)), with none of these mutants mapping to a chromosomal segment homologous with human chromosome 10q where the gene coding for RET (a receptor tyrosine kinase protooncogene) has been localized (Lyonnet *et al.*, 1993).

10 Databases

A very significant effort has been made since the early days of mouse genetics to collect and organize genetic mapping data obtained by all laboratories. The former *Mouse News Letter*, now *Mouse Genome* (Oxford University Press, edited by J. Peters), contains up-to-date information on mouse variants, linkages, inbred strains and nomenclature. It is published as four quarterly issues, each one having a theme: genetic linkage maps and maps of chromosome anomalies; listings of gene symbols and chromosome anomalies; history and location of inbred, congenic and recombinant inbred strains, as well as inter-strain variation; listings of DNA clones, probes, libraries and RFLPs. It also contains short reports from individual laboratories.

More recently, databases have been developed to store and retrieve genetic information and are now available on the Internet. The most concerted effort has been undertaken at the Jackson Laboratory with the development of the Mouse Genome Database (MGD) which aims at making available to the entire scientific community a very large amount of information related to the mouse genome, including mouse locus information, genetic mapping data, mammalian homology data (for over 40 species), probes, clones, PCR primers, genetic polymorphisms, a catalogue of mouse mutations (continuation of the work initiated by Margaret Green), and characteristics of inbred strains. Most of this information is available on-line at the Web site: http://www.informatics.jax.org. MGD is now linked with a set of programs called 'The Encyclopaedia of the Mouse Genome' that enables one to display genetic maps which can be customized. Also available from the same Web sites are the Mouse Chromosome Committee Reports (published annually in *Mammalian Genome* (Springer International), and the most recent maps of the microsatellites cloned by the MIT. A user support service is provided by e-mail to mgi-help@informatics.jax.org.

Another genome database, Mousedb, has been developed at the MRC Radiobiology Unit (Harwell, UK) and is accessible (under X-Windows system only) from the HGMP computing centre (Oxford, UK). It uses the ACeDB database software. Mousedb contains data collated from the published literature only. The data comprise human–mouse homologies including those with pathology, mouse chromosome anomalies, mouse imprinted regions, mouse gene list and data from the *Mouse Chromosome Atlas* maps. The maps are consensus ones based on these data. More information can be obtained by e-mail to r.selley@har-rbu.mrc.ac.uk or kirbym@har-rbu.mrc.ac.uk.

Acknowledgements

We thank Dr Xavier Montagutelli for his contribution to Sections 7 and 10. This work was supported by grants from the Institut Pasteur and the European Union.

References

Bishop, M. (1994). *Guide to Human Genome Computing*. Academic Press, London.

Bonhomme, F., Martin, S. and Thaler, L. (1978). *Experientia* **34**, 1140–1141.

Bonhomme, F. and Guénet, J.-L. (1989). In *Genetic Variants and Strains of the Laboratory Mouse* (M. F. Lyon and A. G. Searle, eds), pp. 649–662. Oxford University Press, Oxford.

Bonhomme, F., Guénet, J.-L., Dod B., Moriwaki, K. and Bulfield G., (1987). *Biol. J. Linn. Soc. Lond.* **30**, 51–58.

Breen, M., Deakin, L., MacDonald, B., Miller, S., Sibson, R., Tarttelin, E., Avner, P., Bourgade, F., Guénet, J.-L., Montagutelli, X., Poirier, C., Simon, D., Tailor, D., Bishop, M., Kelly, M., Rysavy, F., Rastan, S., Norris, D., Shepherd, D., Abbott, C., Pilz, A., Hodge, S., Jackson, I., Boyd, Y., Blair, H., Maslen, G., Todd, J. A., Reed, P. W., Stoye, J., Ashworth, A., McCarthy, L., Cox, R., Schalwyk, L., Lehrach, H., Klose, J., Gangadharan, U. and Brown, S. (1994). *Hum. Mol. Genet.* **3**, 621–627.

Bronson, R. T., Sweet, H. O., Spencer, C. A. and Davisson, M. T. (1992). *J. Neurogenet.* **8**, 71–83.

Bronson, R. T., Lake, B. D., Cook, S., Taylor, S. and Davisson, M. T. (1993). *Ann. Neurol.* **33**, 381–385.

Bueno Brunialti, A. L., Poirier, C., Schmalbruch, H. and Guénet, J.-L. (1995). *Genomics* (in press).

Chalepakis, G., Fritsch, R., Fickenscher, H., Deutsch, U., Goulding, M. and Gruss, P. (1991). *Cell* **66**(5), 873–884.

Copeland, N. G. and Jenkins, N. A. (1991). *Trends Genet.* **7**, 113–118.

Copeland, N. G., Jenkins, N. A., Gilbert, D. J., Eppig, J. T., Maltais, L. J., Miller, J. C., Dietrich, W. F., Weaver, A., Lincoln, S. E., Steen, R. G., Stein, L. D., Nadeau, J. H. and Lander, E. S. (1993). *Science* **262**, 57–66.

Cuénot, L. (1902). *Comptes Rendus de l'Académie des Sciences*.

Dietrich, W., Katz, H., Lincoln, S. E., Shin, H.-S., Friedman, J., Dracopoli, N. C. and Lander, E. S. (1992). *Genetics* **131**, 423–447.

Dietrich, W., Miller, J. C., Steen, R. G., Merchant, M., Damron, D., Nafh, R., Gross, A., Joyce, D. C., Wessel, M., Dredge, R. D., Marquis, A., Stein, L. D., Goodman, N., Page, D. C. and Lander, E.S. (1994). *Nature Genet.* **7**, 220–245.

Gibson, F., Walsh, J., Mburu, P., Varela, A., Brown, K. A., Antonio, M., Beisel, K. W., Steel, K. P. and Brown, S. D. M. (1995). *Nature* **374**, 62–64.

Guénet, J. L., Simon-Chazottes, D. and Avner, P. R. (1988). *Curr. Top. Microbiol. Immunol.* **137**, pp. 13–17.

Haldane, J. B. S., Sprunt, A. D. and Haldane N. M. (1915). *J. Genet.* **5**, 133–135.

Harada, Y., Bonhomme, F., Natsumme-Sakai, S., Tomita, T. and Moriwaki, K. (1989). *Immunogenetics* **29**(3), 148–154.

Hastie, N. D. (1989). In *Genetic Variant and Strains of the Laboratory Mouse* (M. F. Lyon and A. G. Searle, eds), pp. 559–573. Oxford University Press, Oxford.

Hayashizaki, Y., Hirotsune, S., Okazaki, Y., Shibata, H., Akasako, A., Muramatsu, M., Kawai, J., Hirasawa, T., Watanabe, S., Shiroishi, T., Moriwaki, K., Taylor, B. A., Matsuda, Y., Elliott, R. W., Manly, K. F. and Chapman, V. M. (1994). *Genetics* **138**, 1207–1238.

Hearne, C., McAleer, M., Love, J., Aitman, T., Cornall, R., Ghosh, S., Knight, A., Prins, J. B. and Todd, J. (1991). *Mamm. Genome* **1**, 273–282.

Janocha, S., Wolz, W., Srnsen, S., Srsnova, K., Montagutelli, X., Guénet, J.-L., Grimm, T. Kress, W. and Müller, C. M. (1994). *Genomics* **19**, 5–8.

Lander, E. S. and Green, P. (1987). *Proc. Natl. Acad. Sci. USA* **84**, 2363–2367.

Lathrop, G. M. and Lalouel, J. M. (1984). *Am. J. Hum. Genet.,* **36**, 460–465.

Lincoln, S. and Lander, E. (1992). *Genomics* **14**, 604–610.

Lincoln, S., Daly, M. and Lander, E. (1992a). *Constructing Genetic Maps with MAP-MAKER/EXP 3.0.* Whitehead Institute Technical Report, 3rd edn.

Lincoln, S., Daly, M. and Lander, E. (1992b). *Mapping Genes Controlling Quantitative Traits with MAPMAKER/QTL 1.1.* Whitehead Institute Technical Report, 3rd edn.

Love, J. M., Knight, A. M., McAleer, M. A. and Todd, J. (1990). *Nucl. Acid Res.* **18**, 4123–4130.

Lyon, M. F. and Searle, A. G. (1989). *Genetic Variants and Strains of the Laboratory Mouse.* Oxford University Press, Oxford.

Lyonnet, S., Bolino, A., Pelet, A., Abel, L., Nihoul-Fékété, C., Briard, M. L., Mok-Siu, V., Kaariainen, H., Martucciello, G., Lerone, M., Puliti, A., Luo, Y., Weissenbach, J., Devoto, M., Munnich, A. and Romeo, G. (1993). *Nature Genet.* **4**, 346–350.

Mammalian Genome (1994). **5** (special issue).

Manly, K. (1993). *Mamm. Genome* **4**, 303–313.

Matise, T. C., Perlin, M. and Chakravarti, A. (1994). *Nature Genet.* **6**, 384–390.

Montagutelli, X. (1990). *J. Hered.* **81**, 490–491.

Montagutelli, X., Serikawa, T. and Guénet, J. L. (1991). *Mamm. Genome* **1**, 255–259.

Montagutelli, X., Lalouette, A., Coude, M., Kamoun, P., Forest, P. and Guénet, J. L. (1994). *Genomics* **19**, 9–11.

Moore, K. J., Swing, D. A., Rinchik, E. M., Mucenski, M. L., Buchberg, A. M., Copeland, N. G. and Jenkins (1988). *Genetics* **119**(4), 933–941.

Nadeau, J. H., Davinson, M. T., Doolittle, D. P., Grant, P., Hillyard, A. L., Kosowsky, M. and Roderick, H. T. (1992). *Mamm. Genome* **3**, 480–536.

Orita, M., Iwahana, H., Kanazawa, H., Hayashi, K. and Sekiya, T. (1989a). *Proc. Natl. Acad. Sci. USA* **86**, 2766–2770.

Orita, M., Suzuki, Y., Sekiya, T. and Hayashi, K. (1989b). *Genomics* **5**, 874–879.

Schmalbruch, H. M. D., Jensen, H., Bjearg, M., Kamienniecka, Z. and Kurland, B. S. (1991). *J. Neuropath. Exp. Neurol.* **50**, 192–204.

Sendtner, M., Schmalbruch, H., Stockli, K. A., Carroll, P., Kreutzberg, G. W. and Thoenen, H. (1992). *Nature* **358**, 502–504.

Serikawa, T., Montagutelli, M., Simon-Chazottes, D. and Guénet, J.-L. (1992). *Mamm. Genome* **3**, 1992.

Sicinski, P., Geng, Y., Ryder-Cook, A. S., Barnard, E. A., Darlison, M. G. and Barnard, P. J. (1989). *Science* **244**, 1578–1580.

Siracusa, L. D., Jenkins, N. A. and Copeland, N. G. (1991). *Genetics* **127**, 169–179.

Stoye, J. P. and Coffin, J. M. (1988). *J. Virol.* **62**, 168–175.

Taylor, B. A. (1978). In *Origin of Inbred Mice* (H.C. Morse III, ed), pp. 423–438. Academic Press, New York.

Taylor, B. A. and Rowe, L. (1989). *Genomics* **5**, 221–232.

Terwilliger, J. D. and Ott, J. (1992). *Handbook of Human Genetic Linkage*. Johns Hopkins University Press, Baltimore.

Weil, D., Blanchard, S., Kaplan, J., Guilford, P., Gibson, F., Walsh, J., Mburu, P., Varela, A., Levillers, J., Weston, M. D., Kelley, P. M., Kimberling, W. J., Wagenaar, M., Levi-Acobas, F., Larget-Piet, D., Munnich, A., Steel, K. P., Brown, S. D. M. and Petit, C. (1995). *Nature* **374**, 60–61.

Welsh, J., Petersen, C. and McClelland, M. (1991). *Nucl. Acid Res.* **19**, 303–306.

Williams, J. G. K., Kubelik, A. R., Livak, K. J., Rafalski, J. A. and Tingey, S. V. (1990). *Nucl. Acid Res.* **18**, 6531–6535.

Zhang, Y., Proença, R., Maffei, M., Barone, M., Leopold, L. and Friedman, J. M. (1994). *Nature* **372**, 425–432.

II

INTERPRETING THE CODE

4

Exploring the Vast Territory of Uncharted ESTs

JEAN-MICHEL CLAVERIE

CNRS-EP 91, Information Génétique et Moléculaire, IBSM, 31 Chemin Joseph Aiguier, 13402 Marseille Cedex 20, France

Abstract

Large-scale sequencing of partial cDNAs for the generation of expressed sequence tags (ESTs) (Adams *et al.*, 1991) has been proposed as a means to speed up gene discovery (in particular human disease genes) and the identification of new targets for drug development. Current EST projects involve a wide range of evolutionary phyla such as vertebrates (*Homo sapiens, Mus musculus*), invertebrates (*Caenorhabditis elegans*), plants (*Arabidopsis thaliana, Oriza sativa, Zea mays*), yeast and *Plasmodium falciparum*. Until now, most applications have been limited to ESTs displaying significant similarities with already characterized proteins, thus providing a hint about their functions. This, however, corresponds to only 30% of all public ESTs, as shown in the present study.

Characterizing the remaining 70% of 'unknown' ESTs constitutes a major challenge of the Genome Project and for the pharmaceutical application of this kind of data. A first step may be to prioritize the study by trying to identify *a priori* the most promising unknown ESTs. The ESTs exhibiting strong conservation across species and/or constituting families of related genes (paralogs and/or orthologs) constitute a particularly interesting subset.

An inter-species comparison strategy is presented that, despite the redundancy and high noise/signal ratio of EST data, allowed the discovery of 180 new protein families. One hundred and five of these new families are characterized in plants, with 94 of them shared by mono- and dicotyledon angiosperms. These ESTs might characterize a number of 'plant-specific' genes as they do not have homologues in other kingdoms. Fifty-two of the newly discovered families correspond to previously unknown ancient conserved regions (ACRs) (Green *et al.*, 1993; Claverie, 1993a), i.e. sequence segments pre-dating the metazoan radiation, 500–600 million years ago. These are the first representatives of protein families which probably

GENOMES, MOLECULAR BIOLOGY AND DRUG DISCOVERY
ISBN 0-12-137790-3

have a critical but as yet unknown function in a wide range of evolutionary distant organisms.

1 Introduction

Numerous laboratories throughout the world are engaged in the systematic sequencing of the genomes of a wide range of organisms (recently reviewed in Claverie (1995)). The list includes the Gram-negative *Escherichia coli*, the Gram-positive *Bacillus subtilis*, *Mycobacterium leprae*, and *Saccharomyces cerevisiae*, the nematode *Caenorhabditis elegans*, as well as mammals such as humans and mouse. Complete genomic sequences have also been determined for a few large DNA viruses, such as cytomegalovirus and other herpes viruses, vaccinia and variola, Epstein–Barr virus and one baculovirus. Large human genomic sequences have also been determined in the context of the identification of human disease genes by the positional cloning approach (i.e. on the basis of chromosomal location in the absence of prior knowledge about the candidate defective protein).

In the case of human and other mammals, random genomic sequencing is not a cost-effective approach to discovering anonymous protein coding genes due to the large excess of intronic and intergenic segments. Instead, Venter and his co-workers (Adams *et al.*, 1991, 1992, 1993a,b) have proposed the concept of expressed sequences tags (ESTs), i.e. the large-scale characterization of cDNAs from a number of organisms and tissues by the determination of short (300–400 nucleotide), single-pass, partial sequences. This approach has become very popular, and EST sequences have been rapidly accumulated by various public and private laboratories. The main public projects have included human (Adams *et al.*, 1991, 1992, 1993a,b; Okubo *et al.*, 1992; Khan *et al.*, 1992; Grausz and Auffray, 1993), mouse (Davies *et al.*, 1994), *Caenorhabditis elegans* (Waterston *et al.*, 1992), *Arabidopsis thaliana* (Newman, 1993; Desprez *et al.*, 1993), *Oriza sativa* (rice) (Yuzo and Takuji, 1993), and *Plasmodium falciparum* (Reddy *et al.*, 1993; Chakrabarti *et al.*, 1994). Recently, an even larger effort aimed at the determination of 200 000 human EST sequences has begun (sponsored by Merck, under the scientific direction of R. Waterston in St Louis, MO, USA).

The rationale behind EST sequencing is to rapidly elaborate a repertoire of unique mRNA tags for a large fraction of all the genes expressed (yet anonymous) in a given tissue and/or organism. These tags can then be used to speed up the process of gene discovery (i.e. identifying the gene/protein responsible for a given function, a given phenotype or disease state) provided (i) they are assigned to a chromosomal location near a known genetic locus, or (ii) a hint about their function can be derived on the basis of their sequence alone.

While the sequencing has proceeded very rapidly, no map information is yet available for the vast majority of ESTs. Thus, the application of these data has so far been limited to the subset of ESTs with a recognizable sequence similarity to previously characterized genes. Hence, the main utility of the EST approach for the pharmaceutical industry has been in the discovery of new members (e.g. close paralogs) of well-established vertebrate protein families such as cytokines and receptors of neuro-mediators.

2 The fraction of 'unknowns' in genomic and partial cDNA sequences

2.1 The 90%–50% rule

Caenorhabditis elegans and the yeast *Saccharomyces cerevisiae* are the only two organisms for which large new genomic contigs are regularly produced. In yeast, genes interrupted by introns are rare, and protein coding exons can easily be inferred from the analysis of open reading frames (ORF). Introns are more frequent in *C. elegans*, but a significant bias in codon usage and good consensus for the splice sites make the computer identification of exons quite reliable. From the random sampling of protein coding genes newly generated by these two genome projects, one finds that less than 50% have a significant homology with a protein sequence already in databases such as Swiss-Prot (Bairoch and Boeckmann, 1994) or PIR (Barker *et al.*, 1993). Green *et al.* (1993a) and Claverie (1993a) have shown that this result is not due to the incompleteness of the present database. In fact, they have shown that most (90%) of the ancestral protein motifs expected to be shared by most organisms (i.e. predating the metazoan radiation) are indeed represented in the database. The fraction of 50% of 'unknowns' in fact means that (i) only one organism per phylum is currently actively sequenced, and (ii) 50% of the proteins constituting those organisms might in fact be specific to their phylum.

Provided EST sequences from vertebrates represent a random sampling of their protein coding genes, we expect the same argument (the 90%–50% 'rule') to hold. In fact, the presence of 3′ untranslated regions (not expected to resemble any protein) is expected to decrease even further the overall fraction of ESTs displaying a significant similarity in the protein databases.

2.2 Determining the fraction of 'unknown' ESTs

ESTs are short sequences averaging approximately 300 base pairs in length. Local alignment programs of the BLAST family (Altschul *et al.*, 1990) are well suited to search for relatives of such short segments in the databases. In addition, best local alignment algorithms (high score pairing segments (Karlin *et al.*, 1990) or weight matrices (Claverie, 1994b) are mathematically tractable, allowing a measure of statistical significance to be associated with every match. Various implementations of the BLAST algorithm are adapted to a particular query/target database situation: BLASTP for protein/protein sequence comparison, BLASTX for DNA/protein sequence comparison, BLASTN for DNA/DNA sequence comparison, and TBLASTX (Gish, unpublished) for DNA/DNA sequence comparisons using any of their six protein translations.

To identify reliably (even distant) homologues, it is best to translate the EST sequences in all six reading frames and try to match each of them against the protein sequence databases. Searching with protein translations allows the characterization by homology to be carried out to its full potential. If query and target are very similar at the nucleotide level, this will also be indicated by a near perfect match of the conceptual translation. But in many instances, conceptual translations will match significantly in the absence of recognizable similarity of the corresponding DNA sequences. This is what allows the potential function of an EST to be inferred from matches with known protein across highly divergent species, such as human/*C. elegans*, human/yeast (e.g. the discovery of a human homologue of CDC27 (Tugendreich *et al.*, 1993)), or human/*Escherichia coli* (e.g. the hereditary non-polyposis colon cancer MSH2 gene similar to the bacterial mutS mismatch repair protein (Fishel *et al.*, 1993; Leach *et al.*, 1993)).

Unless stated otherwise, we considered BLASTP, BLASTX and TBLASTX similarity scores ≥ 80 as biologically significant. For a random 300-nucleotide DNA sequence, translated in all six frames, and searched against NRDB (NCBI's non-redundant database) using the blosum62 scoring matrix (Henikoff and Henikoff, 1993), the probability of such scores occurring at random is very small ($P < 0.0005$). The target database NRDB is built daily from the non-identical protein sequences derived from GenBank (Benson *et al.*, 1994) coding regions, Swiss-Prot (Bairoch and Boeckmann, 1994) and PIR (Barker *et al.*, 1993). The release we used (November 1994) contained 142 291 sequences of 39 256 841 residues.

Despite the use of a fairly conservative significance threshold, we knew that the results of matching the content of the dbEST database with NRDB (using BLASTX) was going to contain a large fraction of non-biologically significant matches. The artefactual contribution is in fact large enough to make the results clearly dubious: 70% of all ESTs in dbEST are found to match a known protein, a clear violation of the 90%–50% rule we mentioned earlier. The origin of those artefactual matches (see Claverie, 1994a; Claverie and States, 1993, for details) is 2-fold.

(i) Sequences sharing similarly biased composition may generate high similarity scores which do not imply homology (common ancestry). EST nucleotide sequences contain 'simple' segments (e.g. a poly-A tail), which are turned into 'simple' amino acid sequences upon conceptual translation (e.g. poly-K, poly-F). Such segments (Fig. 1) tend to match unrelated proteins exhibiting similarly biased regions.

(ii) Contaminations of both the databases and the EST sequences by vector, ribosomal RNA, Alu repeats (Claverie and Makalowski, 1994), and mitochondrial sequences can also lead to matches with high similarity scores.

The cure to these problems is known and has been presented in detail elsewhere (Claverie and States, 1993; Claverie, 1994a, 1995). It involves the systematic use of 'query masking'. Low entropy segments are easily eliminated using the XNU (Claverie and States, 1993; Claverie, 1994a) and SEG programs (Wootton and Federhen, 1993; Altschul *et al.*, 1994). Sequence contaminations are simply filtered using a preliminary TBLASTX search against an *ad hoc* junk sequence database, the

>sp|P02734|ANP4_PSEAM ANTIFREEZE PEPTIDE 4 PRECURSOR.
    Score= 123, P= 5.7e-12, Identities= 31/38 (81%)

```
Query:     1 AAAAAAAAAAAAAAAAAAAAAAAAAAAAAAAAAAAAAA 38
             AAAAAAA AA AAAAAAA AA AAAAAAA AA AA AA
Sbjct:    27 AAAAAAATAATAAAAAAATAATAAAAAAATAATAAKAA 64
```

>sp|P31231|CAQS_RANES CALSEQUESTRIN, SKELETAL MUSCLE.
    Score= 246, P= 1.3e-26, Identities = 41/41 (100%)

```
Query:     1 DDDDDDDDDDDDDDDDDDDDDDDDDDDDDDDDDDDDDDDDD 41
             DDDDDDDDDDDDDDDDDDDDDDDDDDDDDDDDDDDDDDDDD
Sbjct:   377 DDDDDDDDDDDDDDDDDDDDDDDDDDDDDDDDDDDDDDDDD 417
```

>sp|P19351|TRT_DROME TROPONIN T, SKELETAL MUSCLE
    Score= 169, P= 1.8e-13, Identities= 33/35 (94%),

```
Query:     1 EEEEEEEEEEEEEEEEEEEEEEEEEEEEEEEEEEE 35
             EE+EE+EEEEEEEEEEEEEEEEEEEEEEEEEEEEE
Sbjct:   361 EEDEEDEEEEEEEEEEEEEEEEEEEEEEEEEEEEE 395
```

>sp|P15605|YM04_PARTE HYPOTHETICAL 18.8 KD PROTEIN (ORF4).
    Score= 112, P= 4.6e-13, Identities= 21/41 (51%),

```
Query:     1 FFFFFFFFFFFFFFFFFFFFFFFFFFFFFFFFFFFFFFFFF 41
             FFFF +   FFF FF FF  FF +F +   FFF   F  FFF
Sbjct:    83 FFFFNYLSGFFFLFFVFFTSFFVYFSYLLFFFVPVFVLFFF 123
```

>sp|P29974|CGCC_MOUSE CGMP-GATED CATION CHANNEL PROTEIN
    Score= 137, P= 1.6e-11, Identities= 27/47 (57%),

```
Query:     1 KKKKKKKKKKKKKKKKKKKKKKKKKKKKKKKKKKKKKKKKKKKKKKK 47
             K+KKKKK+KK K   K + K  +KKKK+K+K+KKKK++K K+KK+
Sbjct:    94 KEKKKKKKEKKSKADDKNEIKDPEKKKKKEKEKKKKEEKTKEKKE 140
```

Fig. 1 Example of low entropy matches. These alignments were generated by scanning the protein database with a synthetic query made of homopolymeric segments. Target (real) protein entries with such anomalous sequences (they exist for all but the most hydrophobic residues) cause artefactual matches, mostly to non-coding nucleotide sequences (such as found in genomic and EST sequences). The XNU program was used to mask the low entropy sequences in this study.

result of which is then processed by the XBLAST filter (Claverie and States, 1993; Claverie, 1994a).

In addition, EST sequences with fewer than 100 nucleotides (not counting 'N's or other ambiguities) were also eliminated so as not to artificially inflate the statistics of 'unknowns' (sequences that are too short cannot reach high enough similarity scores).

Finally, we excluded from our analysis EST sequences from libraries for which bacterial or yeast contamination (Savakis and Doelz, 1993) have been reported.

Using the same threshold as before, but with all artefactual contributions removed, the fraction of ESTs with detectable relatives in the protein databases was established at 31% (based on the data from the public dbEST database (Boguski *et al.*, 1993, version 2.9, with 34 091 total entries). A large majority of the accumulated partial cDNA sequence data is thus comprised of 'unknown' ESTs, for which no chromosomal location or functional information is available. In the context of basic research, the unclassified ESTs are the most interesting as they might reveal totally new pathways of cellular metabolism, regulation and communication. Given that this percentage is representative of the situation for all data sets (including proprietary ones), the characterization of these 'unknowns' (e.g. soon to be in the order of 100 000 partial cDNA sequences) becomes a major challenge for the 'post-genome project era'. The next section describes a strategy to prioritize this task.

3   Looking for new protein families in the set of 'unknown' ESTs

3.1   Methods

We will not elaborate further on the above 'classified' EST subset, but, on the contrary, try to characterize the more interesting complementary subset of the 'unknowns', e.g. those exhibiting no convincing match to any known protein or hypothetical ORF.

Without chromosomal location or functional clue, these EST sequences can only be studied in relation to themselves. In this limited context, we can still ask an important biological question: is there evidence of evolutionarily conserved protein families in that set of unknowns? A general strategy to answer this question is to perform an exhaustive search for the presence of clusters of similar putative coding sequences within this set. For this, we used the TBLASTX program (DNA/DNA translation-dependent comparison) to compare all unknown ESTs (e.g. the EST subset complementary to the set of 'known' ESTs delimited by the search described in the preceding section) against each other. This experiment allowed us to partition the unknown ESTs into two categories: (i) the unknown *and* 'unique', exhibiting no significant match to any other unknown EST (irrespective of the species), and (ii) the unknown *but* 'matched'. The relevant numbers are presented in Table 1.

The 'matched' EST subset was then investigated further for the presence of recurrent protein motifs. The 'matched' subset is comprised of both trivial (redundant) and informative similarity clusters. Trivial similarity clusters involve identical (or nearly identical, because of experimental errors) ESTs originating from the same species. In contrast, really informative similarity clusters are those involving ESTs from different species, exhibiting a significant similarity at the protein level.

As a criterion for the automated identification of recurrent, previously unknown, protein motifs, we used the simultaneous requirements of cross-species protein match *and* low similarity at the nucleotide level in our study of the 'matched'

Table 1 Fraction of unknown ESTs (main organisms) in dbEST.v2.9 (33 566 entries >99nt)

	H. sapiens	M. musculus	C. elegans	A. thaliana	O. sativa	Z. mays	P. falciparum
No. genes[a]	85 000	85 000	16 000	20 000	20 000	20 000	7 000
Total ESTs	17 124	374	4 699	5 115	4 341	481	1 104
Known[b]	4 018 (0.23)	66 (0.18)	1 772 (0.38)	2 357 (0.46)	1 802 (0.42)	192 (0.40)	210 (0.19)
Unknown[c]	13 106 (0.77)	308 (0.82)	2 927 (0.62)	2 758 (0.54)	2 539 (0.58)	289 (0.60)	894 (0.81)
Unique[d]	9 588 (0.73)	252 (0.82)	1 663 (0.57)	1 396 (0.51)	1 532 (0.60)	192 (0.66)	689 (0.77)
Matched[e]	3 518	56	1 264	1 362	1 007	97	205

[a]Current estimate.

[b]At least one protein similarity detected (BLASTX + filtering, score ≥ 80, blosum62) against NRDB (163 812 sequences, 35 199 603 residues).

[c]No protein similarity detected (using the previous criteria), total unknown (including species not shown): 23 115, thus 23 115/33 566 = 68.86%. The proportion from total ESTs is in parentheses.

[d]Unknown ESTs *not* matching (TBLASTX + filtering, score ≥ 80, blosum62) any other from any organism. Proportion from unknown EST is in parentheses.

[e]Unknown ESTs matching one or more other unknown ESTs from any organism.

Table 2 Distribution of cross-organism matches

	A. thaliana	O. sativa	H. sapiens	P. falciparum	Z. mays	Capra hircus	C. elegans	M. musculus	Sus. scrofa
A. thaliana	—								
O. sativa	93	—							
H. sapiens	8	18	—						
P. falciparum	5	3	2	—					
Z. mays	11	15	2	1	—				
C. hircus	0	0	4	0	0	—			
C. elegans	11	8	15	2	0	1	—		
M. musculus	0	0	17	0	1	2	1	—	
S. scrofa	0	0	1	0	0	0	0	0	—
Gallus domesticus	0	0	0	0	0	0	0	0	0

These data incorporate the following 3-way, 4-way and 5-way matches:
(H. sapiens/C. hircus/M. musculus), 3× (A. thaliana /O. sativa /Z. mays),
3× (A. thaliana /O. sativa/H. sapiens), 2× (O. sativa/H. sapiens/C. elegans),
(A. thaliana/O. sativa/C. elegans), (O. sativa/H. sapiens/Z. mays),
(A. thaliana/O. sativa/P. falciparum),
2× (A. thaliana/O. sativa/P. falciparum/H. sapiens/C. elegans).

unknown ESTs. This is a powerful criterion given the *a priori* low quality of the EST data (including the possibility of cross-species contamination). Furthermore, we applied this criterion in the most conservative way: we disregarded any cluster of ESTs showing any significant similarity at the nucleotide level.

3.2 Results: 180 new protein families

Table 2 lists the similarity clusters including ESTs from different species (up to four, see legend), with highly significant matches ($P < 0.0005$) at the protein level, and percentage of nucleotide identity usually less than 60% (e.g. not aligned by FASTA (Pearson, W.R., 1990) or BLASTN (score ≤ 110 with the default scoring system, $P > 0.01$).

Figure 2 shows the alignment of two ESTs from *Arabidopsis* and human. This alignment is typical of the matches considered here: two well-conserved amino acid sequences encoded by very divergent nucleotide sequences. Those constraints ensure that the two ESTs are indeed coding regions for two homologous proteins.

This strategy led to the identification of 180 independent EST similarity clusters, each defining a different protein motif common to two or more species. The detail of the cross-species matches defining those clusters is shown in Table 2. In Fig. 3, the same 180 new protein motifs are tentatively positioned on a tree given the evolutionary distance of the organisms involved. It is immediately apparent that, among the newly discovered protein motifs, a minority are identified by matches between ESTs from the most distant phyla in the set. Vertebrate/invertebrate EST matches define 13 of them, plant/animal EST matches define 33 of them, and the six most ancestral motifs are defined by plant or animal ESTs matching with the protozoan *P. falciparum* (Fig. 3). Those instances represent the discovery of 52 new ACRs as originally defined by Green *et al.* (1993).

3.3 Single species paralogs

EST sequence data are plagued by a high error rate. It is usually quite risky to decide that two matching ESTs *from the same species* in fact originate from two distinct, related genes (paralogs), rather than represent variations (allelic or experimental) of the same gene. Still, this ambiguity can be resolved with confidence in the rare cases when two ESTs, while strongly divergent at the nucleotide level, appear to encode very similar amino acid sequences. Such an example in shown in Fig. 4 for two human ESTs and their conceptual translations. Such a strong similarity (47% at the protein level) associated with only 56.5% of identical nucleotides is very unlikely to occur from two inaccurate determinations of the sequence of the same gene. Instead, it is strongly suggestive of two ESTs from paralogous genes. Following this criterion, the pair-wise comparisons of translated ESTs revealed 15 additional new protein motifs defined by paralogous clusters from human, rice and *Arabidopsis*.

```
dbest l 34135 cDNA A.thaliana, 400 nt, rf: +3
dbest l 27681 cDNA H.sapiens, 399 nt, rf: +3    Similarity score: 280

34135: 102  DDNDVDLRLARLEELMNRRPALANSVLLRQNPHNVEQWHRRVKIFEGNSAKQILTYTEAV 281
            DD D++LRLAR E+L +RRP L NSVLLRQNPH+V +WH+RV + +G    + I TYTEAV
27681:  66  DDVDLELRLARXEQLXSRRPLLINSVLLRQNPHHVHEWHKRVALHQGRPREIINTYTEAV 245

34135: 282  RTXDPMKAVXKPHTXWVAFATLYVNHKDLVNTR 380
            +T DP KA  KPHT WVAF   Y ++  L + R
27681: 246  QTVDPXKATGKPHTLWVAFXKFYXDNGQLDDAR 344


34135: GAT GTT AAT GAT CTG AGA TTG GCT CGT TTG GAA GAA CTG ATG AAC AGA AGA CCT
27681: ... ... GTG ..C C... ..G ... C.C C... ..C ..N .. .G C.G ..C N.C .G. C.G C.G ..C
34135: GCA CTG GCA AAC AGT GTG CTC CTT AGG CAG AAT CCT CAC AAT GTT GAG CAA TGG CAT CGT
27681: CTG ..N CTC ... ..C ..C T.G ..G C.C ..A ... C.C ..A ... C.C ..G C.C G.G ... .. ..C AAG
34135: AGA GTC AAA ATA TTT GAG GGA AAC TCA GCA AAG CAG ATT CTC ACA TAC ACA GAA GCA GTG
27681: C.T ... GCC C.G CAC C... ..C CG. C.C CGG G.. ATC ..C AA. ..C ... ... ..G ..T ..N
34135: AGG ACT NTT GAT CCN ATG AAA GCA GTT NGG AAG CCT CAC ACC TTN TGG GTT GCT TTT GCC
27681: CA.. ..G G.G ..C ..C T.N ..G ..C ACA G.C ... ..C ... ..T C... ... ..G ..G ..:. N..
34135: ACG TTG TAT GTA AAC CAC AAA GAC CTC GTC AAT ACT AGG
27681: .A. ..T ... NAG G.. A. GG. C.G .A. G.. G.C C.T
```

Fig. 2 Example of match between two ESTs from very distant organisms, *H. sapiens* and *A. thaliana*. Top: amino acid alignment, showing 57% of identical residues. Bottom: nucleotide alignment of the same segments showing 59% of identical nucleotides (non-identical positions are indicated for EST27681).

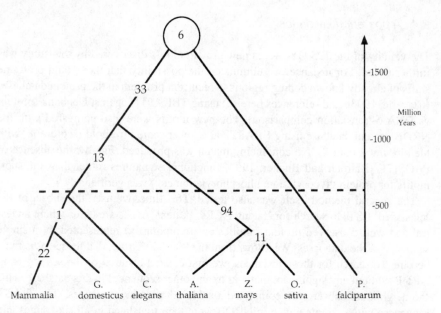

Fig. 3 Putative evolutionary ancestry of the 180 new gene families. Divergence times (in millions of years) are tentative. The dashed line corresponds to the metazoan ancestral conserved region threshold.

```
dbest I 30599  cDNA H.sapiens, 337 nt, rf: -3
dbest I 38993  cDNA H.sapiens, 248 nt, rf: +2  Similarity score: 196 (47% a.a. identity)
```

Putative coding similarity:

```
30599:    320 RRTRSFVAEGLFYNEDNKEDPMSAYFLQFDHLDSEWLGMPPLPSPRCLFGLGEALNSIYVVGGREIK 120
              ++ + +V  GL+ +E+NK+ P+ +YF Q D + SEW+G+PPLPS RCL GLGE  + IYVV G++++
38993:      8 QQNQIYVVGGLYVDEENKDQPLQSYFFQLDSIASEWVGLPPLPSARCLXGLGEVDDKIYVVAGKDLQ 208
```

Corresponding DNA alignment (56.5% nucleotide identity):

```
30599: agg aga acc agg tcc ttc gtg gct gaa ggn ctc ttc tac aac gaa gac aac aaa gag gac
38993: ca. ca. .at ca. ata .at ... .ta .g. ..a ..a .at gtg g.t ... ..a ..t ..g ..t c.a

30599: ccc atg agc gca tac ttc ctg cag ttt gac cat ctg gac tca gag tgg ctg ggg atg cca
38993: ..t c.a cag t.. ... ... t.c ... c.c ..t agc a.a .ca ..t ..a ... g.t ..a c.t ...

30599: ccg ctg ccc tcg ccc cgc tgc ctc ttt ggc ctg gga gaa gct ctc aac tcc atc tac gtg
38993: ..t ... ..t ..a g.. a.g ..t ... .nc ..t ... ... ..g .tg gat g.t aaa ... ..t ..a

30599: gtc ggt ggc aga gag atc aag
38993: ..t .ca ... .a. ..c c.t c.a
```

Fig. 4 Example of human paralogs. The conceptual translations of these two human ESTs exhibit 47% of identical residues, and the corresponding nucleotides are 56.5% identical. A nucleotide sequence divergence that high is unlikely to come from sequencing errors (approx. 1%) or allelic variations. However, the low quality of single-pass sequences does not allow closer paralogous sequences to be discriminated from badly sequenced, EST duplicates.

3.4 A posteriori validation

The validity of the 195 (180 + 15) new protein motifs discovered by this study was further tested. For instance, we eliminated the possibility that they could be frame shifts of already known coding regions (a recurrent problem in the protein databases (Claverie, 1993b and references herein)) using TBLASTN against Genbank (protein vs DNA 6-translation comparison). The new motifs were also compared with the NRDB protein database using BLASTP at a lower score threshold (score ≥68, with the blosum62 matrix). No convincing match was produced. Finally, the absence of PROSITE (Bairoch and Bucher, 1994) functional signatures (other than the short motifs for protein glycosylation, phosphorylation etc.) was verified.

The general method itself was also tested. This time, we used the subset of the 'classified' ESTs to search for 'latent' ACRs. 'Latent' ACRs are cases where ancestral and well-conserved protein families are (temporarily) represented by a single sequence in the databases. We know, from the 90%–50% rule, that those cases must be rare. To search for those instances, we first created a subset of the sequences in NRDB without any significant matches to any other sequences in this database. This 'no-neighbour' subset was comprised of 11 953 protein sequences. The dbEST sequences *with a single match* in NRDB were then translated in all six frames and compared against the 'no-neighbour' set using BLASTX. After discarding the artefactual matches (induced by repeats, frame shifts etc.), this analysis revealed nine latent ACRs. Only one is a protein associated to a known function, ε-COP (Rothman and Orci, 1992). The various COP proteins (α, β, δ, γ, ε and ζ-COP) form the subunits of the coatomer complex in nonclathrin-coated vesicles, involved in intracellular protein trafficking. This is a basic cellular function and, as a consequence, we expect the sequences of the various COP proteins to be themselves conserved in very distant organisms. Figure 5 shows how the bovine ε-COP protein sequence (with no relative in the protein databases) is partially matched by four different ESTs from human, nematode, *Arabidopsis*, and rice. Although each of the ESTs shares a strong sequence similarity with ε-COP, they do not all overlap with each other. Thus, the four ESTs matching ε-COP might define a single ACR, although they form two non-overlapping similarity clusters. Three of the nine additional ACRs were found in proteins of unknown function but isolated in a particular biological context: a rice protein putatively related to chilling tolerance (Binh and Oono, 1992), a 43 kD protein encoded by an abundant transcript in *Drosophila* embryos (unpublished, Oliveri, Banga and Boyd, direct Genbank submission, accession: L01790 1992), and a growth factor responsive gene isolated from vascular smooth muscle cells (Wax *et al.*, 1994). The remaining five new ACR classes are defined by an EST matching conceptual translation of anonymous open reading frames in the genome of yeast (Dujon *et al.*, 1994) or *C. elegans* (Wilson *et al.*, 1994).

```
Human:    9 MAPPAPGPASGGSGXVDELFDVKNAFYIGSYQQCINXAXGXKLSSPERDVFLYRAY
            ||||||||||||| ||||||||||||||||||| | | ||| ||||||||||||||
ε-COP:    1 MAPPAPGPASGGSGEVDELFDVKNAFYIGSYQQCINEAQRVKPSSPERDVFLYRAY
                                                      ++ + +
Rice:                                             81 ERDAIVFRSY


Human:  189 LAQRKFGVVLDEIKPXSAPKLQAVRMFXDYLAHXSRRDSIVAELDREMSRSVDVTNNTF 365
            ||||| |||||||| +||| ||||||| ||||| +|||||||||||||||||||||||
ε-COP:      LAQRKYGVVLDEIKPSSAPELQAVRMFAEYLASHSRRDAIVAELDREMSRSVDVTNTTFL  TF
            +  +|+   | || ||| +++    ||+
Rice:   206 VALGSYQLVISEIDSSAATSLQAVKLLALYLS


thaliana:  4 MQQIDEDHT
             || ||||
ε-COP:       LMAAASIYFYDQNPDAALRTLHQGDSLECMAMTVQILLKLDRLDLARKELKKMQDQDEDAT


thaliana:  LTQLASAWXNLAVGGSKIQEAYLIFQDFSEKYPMTSLILNGKAVCCMHMGNFEEAETLLL 183
           |||||| ||| +|| ||| |+|+||+   | |++ | || ||+ || +++++
ε-COP:     LTQLATAWVSLAAGGEKLQDAYYIFQEMADKCSPTLLLLNGQAACHMAQGRWEAAAEGVLQ
                             + ||| +|| +
C.elegans: 327 YAAAEELLE


thaliana:  EALNKDAKDPETLANLVVCSLHVGK 183
           ||| |+  + |||| | | | +||
ε-COP:     EALDKDSGHPETLINLVLSQHLGKPPEVTNRYLSQLKDAHRSHPFIKEYRAKENDFDRLVLQYAPSA 308
              ||+ +  + +| + || + +    + ||  + | +++ ++ ++| ||+ +||||+
C.elegans: SALERDNKDADVLINSIVSAQLNEKDDDVVERFISQLKHEHPNHPWVIDFNEKEAEFDRV 121
```

Fig. 5 Cross-phylum relative of the bovine ε-COP protein in dbEST. The *Bos taurus* ε-COP protein sequence (in italics) is locally aligned with four matching EST translations. Similar amino acids according to the blosum62 scoring matrix are denoted by '+'. Human EST H1BBJ23 and rice EST C0604A match in the N-terminal region, *A. thaliana* EST 47C12T7 in the middle, and *C. elegans* EST 01216 in the C-terminal region. Percentages of DNA identity for the aligned segments are: 52% with *C. elegans*, 60% with rice, 61% with *A. thaliana*, and 85% with human.

4 Discussion

Starting from 23 115 unclassified ESTs, this study revealed 180 new protein sequence motifs. These new motifs are detected in two or more species and correspond to segments of well-conserved amino acids encoded by nucleotide sequences with little similarity. One hundred and five of these new motifs (more than half) are found in plants, and 94 of them predate the divergence of monocotyledons from the bulk of the other angiosperms, 90–130 million years ago (reviewed in Crane *et al.*, 1995). Those motifs might characterize a number of plant-specific genes as they have not yet been detected in other kingdoms.

The new motifs also include 52 new ACRs as previously defined by Green *et al.* (1993), i.e. conserved sequence motifs predating the coelomate radiation, 500–600 million years ago. Vertebrate/invertebrate matches defined 13 of them, plant/animal matches defined 33, and *Plasmodium*/animal or *Plasmodium*/plant matches defined six. Since ESTs are partial cDNA sequences, some of the similarity clusters defining different motifs might, in fact, correspond to non-overlapping regions of a single unknown protein. This situation was actually seen with the ESTs matching the ε-COP protein (Fig. 5). Thus, fewer than 180 new protein families and less than 52 distinct ACRs might correspond to the results presented here. Since a small number of new ACRs remain to be found, similarity clusters of ESTs corresponding to different segments of the same unknown ancestral protein are expected to occur more often. Fifty-two might thus be an overestimate of the truly distinct ancestral protein revealed in this study. We may still use this number to estimate how many ACRs (sampled using the EST approach) are left to be found in the future. In this study, the number of distinct ACRs discovered among the mammalian ESTs is 41, 33 were discovered among the *C. elegans* ESTs, and 17 were common to both mammals and *C. elegans*. These numbers already indicate quite intuitively that we are sampling from a small 'pot' since the fraction of common 'draws' is very large. We can make a quantitative estimate of what is left in the pot using a maximum likelihood approach. Let us denote N = number of metazoan ACRs sampled from the ESTs in this analysis, A = number of mammalian ACRs, B = number of *C. elegans* ACRs and C = number of shared ACRs. Given N, A, and B, the probability, P, of the overlap containing C members is given by:

$$P(C|N,A,B) = \frac{\dfrac{N!}{C!(A-C)!(B-C)!(N-A-B+C)!}}{\dfrac{N!}{A!(N-A)!}\dfrac{N!}{B!(N-B)!}}$$

Given $A = 41, B = 33$ and $C = 17$:

$$P(17 \mid N, 41, 33) = \frac{\dfrac{N!}{17!24!16!(N-57)!}}{\dfrac{N!}{41!(N-41)!} \quad \dfrac{N!}{33!(N-33)!}}$$

Maximizing this ratio gives a maximum likelihood estimation for N, $N_{p(A \cap B = 17)max} \cong 82$. Including the 52 new ACRs found in the present study, this suggests that approximately 30 metazoan ACRs remain to be discovered through the EST approach. Both this result and the small number of new ACRs yielded by the comparison of more than 23 000 unclassified ESTs are consistent with our earlier findings (Green *et al.*, 1993; Claverie, 1993a) that there are relatively few conserved protein classes, probably less than 1000, and that most of them are already represented in the databases.

For the last two decades, most genes were sequenced after the encoded proteins were associated with a particular enzymatic activity, cellular function or physiological process. Then, a purely genetic approach in model organisms, and more recently in humans, allowed the isolation of genes prior to isolation of the encoded proteins. Most recently, large-scale genomic sequencing, as well as the EST approach, has begun to produce large numbers of anonymous gene sequences. We have determined here that less than one-third of the public ESTs bear a significant homology with genes of known function. For the remaining two-thirds of unknown ESTs (soon to amount to more than 100 000 sequences for human) individual functional and/or mapping studies appear unavoidable. Using the public data available in dbEST, we have applied the concept of evolutionary conservation to prioritize this overwhelming task. This approach successfully identified a number of highly conserved, yet unknown, gene families. Most are likely to represent entirely new classes of enzymes, hormones, receptors or transcription factors, and as such, could be promising targets for the biotechnology and pharmaceutical industry.

Acknowledgements

I thank W. Gish for early access to the TBLASTX program, and J. Spouge and J. Wilbur for mathematical advice. The approach and results presented here remain valid despite the very large increase in EST data in recent months.

References

Adams, M. D., Kelley, J. M., Gocayne, J. D., Dubnick, M., Polymeropoulos, M. H., Xiao, H., Merril, C. R., Wu, A., Olde, B., Moreno, R. F. *et al.* (1991). *Science* **252**, 1651–1656.

Adams, M. D., Dubnick, M., Kerlavage, A. R., Moreno, R. F., Kelley, J. M., Utterback, T. R., Nagle, J. W., Fields, C. A. and Venter, J. C. (1992). *Nature* **355**, 632–634.

Adams, M. D., Kerlavage, A. R., Fields, C. and Venter, J. C. (1993a). *Nature Genet.* **4**, 256–267.

Adams, M. D., Soares, M. B., Kerlavage, A. R., Fields, C. and Venter, J. C. (1993b). *Nature Genet.* **4**, 373–380.

Altschul, S. F., Gish, W., Miller, W., Myers, E. W. and Lipman, D. J. (1990). *J. Mol. Biol.* **215**, 403–410.

Altschul, S. F., Boguski, M. S., Gish, W. and Wootton, J. C. (1994). *Nature Genet.* **6**, 119–129.

Bairoch, A. and Boeckmann, B. (1994). *Nucl. Acid Res.* **22**, 3578–3580.

Bairoch, A. and Bucher, P., (1994). *Nucl. Acid Res.* **22**, 3583–3589.

Barker, W. C., George, D. G., Mewes, H.-W., Pfeiffer, F. and Tsugita, A. (1993). *Nucl. Acid Res.* **21**, 3089–3092.

Benson, D. A., Boguski, M., Lipman, D.J. and Ostell, J. (1994). *Nucleic Acid Res.* **22**, 3441–3444.

Binh, L. and Oono, K. (1992). *Plant Physiol.* **99**, 1146–1150.

Boguski, M. S., Lowe, T. M. and Tolstoshev, C. M. (1993). *Nature Genet.* **4**, 332–333.

Chakrabarti, D., Reddy, G. R., Dame, J. B., Almira, E. C., Laipis, P. J., Ferl, R. J., Yang, T. P., Rowe, T. C. and Schuster, S. M. (1994). *Mol. Biochem. Parasitol.* **66**, 97–104.

Claverie, J.-M. (1993a). *Nature* **364**, 19–20.

Claverie, J.-M. (1993b). *J. Mol. Biol.* **234**, 1140–1157.

Claverie, J.-M. (1994a). In *Automated DNA Sequencing and Analysis Techniques* (M.D. Adams, C. Fields and J. C. Venter, eds), Ch. 36, pp. 267–279. Academic Press, New York.

Claverie, J.-M. (1994b). *Comput. Chem.* **18**, 287–294.

Claverie, J.-M. (1995).In *Advances in Computational Biology* (H. Villar, ed.). Jai Press Inc., Greenwicht, CT.

Claverie, J. M. and Makalowski, W. (1994). *Nature* **371**, 752.

Claverie, J. M. and States, D. (1993). *Comput. Chem.* **17**, 191–201.

Crane, P. R., Friis, E. M. and Pedersen, K. R. (1995). *Nature* **374**, 27–33.

Davies, R. W., Roberts, A. B., Morris, A. J., Griffith, G., Jerecic, J., Ghandi, S., Kaiser, K., and Savioz, A. (1994). Direct submission to Genbank (August 1994).

Desprez, T., Amselem, J., Chiapello, H., Caboche, M. and Hofte, H. (1993). Direct submission to GenBank (August 1993).

Dujon, B. *et al.* (1994). *Nature* **369**, 371–378.

Fishel, R. *et al.* (1993). *Cell* **75**, 1027–1038.

Grausz, J.D. and Auffray, C., (1993). *Genomics* **17**, 530–532.

Green, P., Lipman, D., Hillier, L., Waterston, R., States, D. and Claverie, J.-M. (1993). *Science* **259**, 1711–1716.

Henikoff, S. and Henikoff, J. G. (1993). *Proteins* **17**, 49–61.

Karlin, S., Dembo, A. and Kawabata, T. (1990). *Ann. Stat.* **18**, 571–581.

Khan, A. S., Wilcox, A. S., Polymeropoulos, M. H., Hopkins, J. A., Stevens, T. J., Robinson, M., Orpana, A. K. and Sikela, J. M. (1992). *Nature Genet.* **2**, 180–185.

Leach, F. S. *et al.* (1993). *Cell* **75**, 1215–1225.

Newman, T. (1993). Direct submission to GenBank.

Okubo, K., Hori, N., Matoba, R., Niiyama, T., Fukushima, A., Kojima, Y. and Matsubara, K. (1992). *Nature Genet.* **2**, 173–179.

Reddy, G. R., Chakrabarti, D., Schuster, S. M., Ferl, R. J., Almira, E. C. and Dame, J. B. (1993). *Proc. Natl. Acad. Sci. USA* **90**, 9867–9871.

Rothman, J. E. and Orci, L. (1992). *Nature* **355**, 409–415

Savakis, C. and Doelz, R. (1993). *Science* **259**, 1677–1678.

Tugendreich, S., Boguski, M. S., Seldin, M. S. and Hieter, P. (1993). *Proc. Natl. Acad. Sci. USA* **90**, 10031–10005.

Waterston, R., Martin, C., Craxton, M., Huynh, C., Coulson, A., Hillier, L., Durbin, R. K., Green, P., Shownkeen, R., Halloran, N., Hawkins, T., Wilson, R., Berks, M., Du, Z., Thomas, K., Thierry-Mieg, J. and Sulston, J. (1992). *Nature Genet.* **1**, 114–123.

Wax, S. D., Rosenfield, C.L. and Taubman, M. B. (1994). *J. Biol. Chem.* **269**, 13041–13047 .

Wilson, R. *et al.* (1994). *Nature* **368**, 32–38.

Wootton, J. C. and Federhen, S. (1993). *Comput. Chem.* **17**, 149–163.

Yuzo, M. and Takuji, S. (1993). Direct submission to GenBank (November 1993).

5

Prediction of Protein Structures and their Docking

PAUL A. BATES, RICHARD M. JACKSON
and MICHAEL J. E. STERNBERG

Biomolecular Modelling Laboratory, Imperial Cancer Research Fund, 44 Lincoln's Inn Fields, London WC2A 3PX, UK

Abstract

The rapid expansion in the number of sequenced genes has emphasized the need to obtain structural predictions for these proteins and their interactions as a major step on the path to drug design and discovery.

The most powerful method of protein structure prediction relies on identifying that a molecule of unsolved structure resembles a known protein structure. This approach is most accurate when there is a clear sequence homology between the unknown and the known structures. The application of homology modelling is described in the context of our studies of modelling carcinoembryonic antigen (CEA), a colorectal tumour marker that is a member of the immunoglobulin super-family, and of monoclonal antibody PR1A3 that has a markedly increased specificity for CEA attached to tumour cells. The role of modelling to suggest mutational studies is reported.

Recently, a major development in protein structure prediction has been to identify the similarity of protein folds in the absence of sequence similarities detectable from analysis of the primary structure alone. The present status of these threading algorithms is reported.

With the structures of two proteins obtained either experimentally or via prediction, another major computation challenge is to predict their docked conformation. Several approaches are available to generate a set of favourable docked associations and the main difficulty lies in distinguishing the correct docking from a limited set of seemingly equally favourable associations. Recent work on quantifying the hydrophobic effect and the inclusion of both electrostatic desolvation and interaction provides an approach to solve this screening problem. We have recently predicted the docking of β-lactamase and its inhibitor to 2.1 Å accuracy

GENOMES, MOLECULAR BIOLOGY AND DRUG DISCOVERY
ISBN 0-12-137790-3

from the coordinates of the unbound proteins without prior knowledge of the crystallographic complex. If other trials are successful, then computing methods will be able to model protein docking in the absence of large-scale conformational changes.

1 Introduction

Knowledge of the three-dimensional structure of a protein can yield a wealth of information about its mode of action and can direct the systematic design of pharmaceutical agents. Thus many protein structure determinations have had a major impact on medical science (e.g. Perutz, 1992). However despite improvements in protein structure determination by both crystallography and nuclear magnetic resonance, there remains a vast disparity between the number of determined sequences (more than 40 000 in SWISSPROT in 1994 (Bairoch and Boeckmann, 1991)) and the number of solved structures (about 4000 in the Protein databank in 1994 (Bernstein *et al.*, 1977)). This disparity remains after removing proteins with 30% sequence identity to estimate some 9000 non-homologous sequences and 500 non-homologous structures (Orengo *et al.*, 1994). From renaturation experiments the principle that protein sequence determines protein structure in a given environment remains a viable hypothesis motivating the development of algorithms for protein structure prediction.

The most powerful approach for protein structure prediction is to use knowledge, both structural and thermodynamic, obtained from the known protein structures rather than to rely on a search for a minimum energy conformation from interatomic potentials. Figure 1 summarizes the key steps followed to obtain a structural model from a newly determined sequence. This chapter will summarize aspects of this approach for structure prediction.

Structural knowledge of biomolecular interactions is central to understanding and regulating activity. However, sometimes the structures of the components but not the complex are available. Another major challenge is to develop computer algorithms to predict the docking (of two or more) molecules. Any algorithm must at least be able to model the small conformational changes that will always occur on molecular association. We describe here the developments of a docking algorithm that includes the capacity to model the association of accurately predicted protein structure (e.g. docking a predicted antibody against an experimentally determined antigen).

2 Model building by homology

Whenever a new protein sequence is determined, the first step is to search sequence databases to identify homologous sequences. Sometimes a homology is detected with a protein of known three-dimensional structure. Knowledge from the determined structures of families of homologous proteins shows that they have a conserved common core mainly formed from secondary structures with most of the

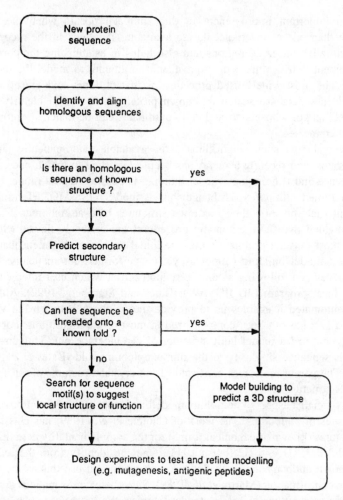

Fig. 1 A flow chart of the approach followed to predict protein structure from sequence.

structural variations occurring in the loop regions. Thus the approach of modelling by homology has proved a powerful and widely used strategy in determining protein structures (e.g. see Blundell *et al.*, 1987; Bates and Sternberg, 1992).

The method involves the following stages.

(i) Align the sequence of unknown structure with parent template structure.

(ii) Identify regions of parent structure that will be structurally conserved in the unknown structure.

(iii) Replace side chains of parent structure in these conserved regions with those of the unknown structure.

(iv) Identify suitable loop conformations for the unknown structure.

(v) Inspect and adjust side chain angles to most favourable conformation.

An important improvement in this approach occurs when the structures of more than one parent molecule are available. This aids in the recognition of the structurally conserved regions and also helps in establishing the correct sequence alignment. Various methods are available to attempt to model the loop conformation. The most widely used procedure is that of Jones and Thirup (1986) which involves a database search of known protein structures to identify loops of the correct length whose start and end coordinates can be matched onto the segments to be connected.

Several of such algorithms are available automatically in modelling programs, and recently a server has been established to which one can mail one's sequence and if homology model building is possible then a model built structure is returned (http://expasy.hcuge.ch/swissmod/SWISS-MODEL.html). However recent trials on modelling unknown structures held at Asilomar, California have highlighted that these automatic procedures are seriously flawed (Shortle, 1995). The most difficult problem is that the initial sequence alignment that is crucial to correct model building cannot as yet be performed automatically. In our group we have been following a combined approach in which user intervention is added to a local program (3D-JIGSAW) (Bates and Sternberg, 1992). Although this is not automated it enables us to provide the feedback between the various stages that as yet has not been computerized in most of the algorithms. For example, we have obtained a model built structure of carcinoembryonic antigen (CEA) based on its sequence similarity to the immunoglobulin fold (Bates *et al.*, 1992) (Plate 1a). The parent molecules consisted of the crystal structures of REI, CD4 and the NMR structure of CD2.

A specialist aspect of homology modelling is that of the prediction of the combining sites of antibodies. The work of Chothia *et al.* (1989) has classified common structures (known as canonical forms) for the complementarity determining loops of L1, L2, L3, H1 and H2 (but not H3). One can identify from the sequence of the unknown antibody the likely loop conformation and use this as the starting main chain conformation (Martin *et al.*, 1989). Side chain conformations are modelled by energy calculations or set to standard angles. We have used such an approach to model the predicted structure of a monoclonal antibody, PR1A3 against CEA (Plate 1b). Inspection of the antigen binding region identifies two glutamic acid residues ideally poised to interact with the antigen. Inspection of the domain of CEA that is identified by PR1A3 identified positively charged Lys residues that could salt bridge to these glutamic acids. Mutagenesis identified that the change of Lys to Ala abolished binding. Thus these model building studies are able to suggest possible antigen/antibody interactions as a first step to altering possible associations. In addition, predicted antibody structures are a powerful guide in humanizing antibodies or in the development of single chain antibodies by the introduction of suitable disulphide cross-links.

3 Protein fold recognition

With the increase in number of known protein structures, it is apparent that proteins that do not possess a sequence similarity which would be detected by sequence searches alone can still adopt a common three-dimensional fold. The current challenge is, given a new sequence, to determine whether it will adopt one of the determined three-dimensional folds. This approach was pioneered by the groups of Eisenberg (Bowie *et al.*, 1991) and Thornton (Jones *et al.*, 1992).

We are developing a program (FoldID) based on the concept that the key feature of fold conservation is a common arrangement of packed secondary structures (Fig. 2). The first step is to use a dynamic programming algorithm to align the probe sequence, denoted p (whose structure one wishes to predict) against each member of a database of known folds (a target fold, denoted t). The scoring function for each cell in the dynamic programming matrix represents a match of one residue of the probe with one residue of target. The function evaluates a match at three levels: primary sequence, secondary structure and tertiary structure. We use information from a series of homologous sequences to improve the matching at the primary and secondary structure stages. The starting point is a multiple sequence alignment that is performed using the PhD file server at Heidelberg (http://www. embl–heidelberg.de/predictprotein/predictprotein.html) established by Rost and Sander (1993). This provides both an alignment of homologous sequences and then uses this information to perform a secondary structure prediction that typically is of 70% accuracy (probably the best available algorithm today). A predicted tertiary profile is based on the scoring scheme of Nishikawa and Ooi (1980) and is an indication of the likelihood of certain residue types to form contacts within the core of the protein.

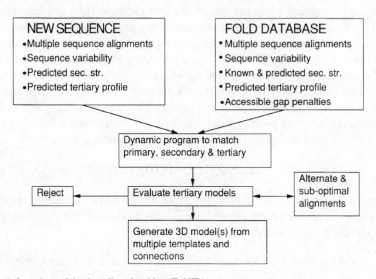

Fig. 2 A flow chart of the threading algorithm (FoldID).

Thus,

cell_score(p,t) =

$W1(Vp \times Vt \times SEQmat) + W2(Cssp \times Csst \times SSmat) + W3(TERTp-TERTt)$

where $W1$, $W2$ and $W3$ are weights currently set at 1.0,
SEQmat is the standard Dayhoff PAM250 matrix (Dayhoff, 1978),
Vp and Vt are the variability of the multiple sequence alignments of p and t,
Cssp and Csst are the confidence levels of the secondary structure prediction obtained from the PhD algorithm,
SSmat is a matrix that quantifies the agreement between the predicted secondary structure of the probe and both the known and predicted secondary structure of the target,
TERTp−TERTt is the difference in the tertiary profiles.

To perform these calculations, a database of known folds is established that contains the multiple sequence alignments, the sequence variability at each position, the X-ray and the predicted secondary structure, and the predicted tertiary contact profile. Associated with each secondary structure of the target folds is a gap penalty used in the dynamic programming algorithm that models the tendency for insertions and deletions in folds to occur in loop regions and in secondary structures that have limited contributions to the tertiary fold. Given a new sequence, the multiple sequence alignment is performed, leading to identification of sequence variability, the predicted secondary structure and the predicted tertiary profile.

The standard dynamic programming algorithm is used to take the new sequence with its associated information and match it at the primary, secondary and tertiary scoring levels against each member of the fold database. The optimal path score based on summing cell scores and subtracting the gap penalties is evaluated using the standard procedure. The final tertiary model score is then obtained and evaluated using two functions. The first (POT) is an indication of pairwise favourable potentials between residues. This is based on observed frequencies of residue–residue interactions between defined secondary structure elements (e.g. the frequency a Leu in a β-strand packs against an Ile in an α-helix). This scoring scheme thus evaluates the secondary structure packing that is the dominant feature of the fold. The second term (POLAR) is a measure of the exposure of polar residues. Thus,

$$final\_score = path\_score \times (POTp - POTt) \times (POLARp - POLARt)$$

Runs of the probe against each target in the database yield a distribution of final scores. Each final score is then scaled to a Z-score to estimate the significance of its value relative to the database:

$$Z\text{-score (target } i) = \frac{\text{final score (target } i) - \text{mean of all target scores}}{\text{standard deviation of all target scores}}$$

Results of trials using known structures that match a member of the fold library are shown in Table 1. The proteins used in this table were based on the published work of Jones *et al.* (1992) to provide a comparison of the success of the algorithms. Our results in terms of position of the correct fold at the top of the list are comparable. Both algorithms identify the proteins that have a common fold but do not have a level of sequence identity that would be identified in a conventional search. Examples of the Z-scores for two of the probes are shown in Fig. 3.

Table 1 also evaluates the accuracy of the equivalences. If the fold prediction is to be used to build a tertiary structure, it is necessary that the residues are correctly equivalenced between the probe and the target fold. Alignments on a residue accuracy are still at a low level. However it must be noted that even with homologous sequences of high sequence relationship automatic methods would not yield a per cent N that is 100% (Barton and Sternberg, 1987). We also evaluate, by inspection, the percentage of secondary structures that are correctly equivalenced. Provided there is high 50% overlap between the secondary structures of the probe and the matched template, we say the secondary structures have been correctly equivalenced. This suggests to what extent an approximate fold could be constructed. Such folds would still be helpful in identifying spatially similar regions as might constitute a discontinuous epitope or might contribute to forming an active site. We have also examined %N and %SS from the recently available programme implementing the algorithm of Jones *et al.* We find that for most our examples the %N and %SS are higher than those of the Jones algorithm.

Clearly the improvement of the alignment in fold recognition is an area for further research and here we wish to highlight that in evaluating any algorithm it is important both to ensure that the correct fold is at the top of the list and that accurate equivalences are obtained. We envisage generating a series of alternate alignments (e.g. by variation of the weights $W1$, $W2$ and $W3$) and screening the tertiary structures that would be generated.

4 Protein docking

The protein docking problem is one of predicting the mode of association of two proteins of unbound conformation. Our initial test system was to model the docking of three monoclonal antibodies to hen lysozyme and to reproduce the crystallographically determined results. Our aim was to develop an algorithm with sufficiently soft potentials to cope not only with the conformational changes on docking but also to be able to dock a predicted antibody structure, given the accuracy of predicting antibody combining sites.

The algorithm, implemented in a program DAPMATCH, was to perform a global search to guarantee generating the correct docking and thereby reduce the problem to one of screening (Walls and Sternberg, 1992). The entire surface of the antigen and the combining site of the antibody are represented as a series of slices of the protein surface. Each slice details the van der Waals surface of the protein over a 32 Å by 32 Å region. The surfaces of the proteins are smooth and represented as a

Table 1 Results of fold identification using FoldID. The probe and its correct fold were scanned against 119 other folds in the database. The top match (second match for run 5) was a protein with the same fold. Other related folds were also found at different positions in the list. The % sequence ID indicates the difficulty of fold recognition. Above 20% would easily be detected by standard homology searches whilst below 15% is unlikely to be identified from sequence alone. The r.m.s fit (of superposable Cα atoms) indicates the similarity between the three-dimensional structures of the probe and best match. Z-score, %N and %SS are given in the text. Note that several aspects of the algorithm need to be cross-validated. The secondary structure prediction uses information about the structure of probe. The tertiary contacts were calculated including the probe. The simplest approach for validation would be blind tests

Probe	Fold	Top of list match	Top of list fold	Other related folds in list	% Seq ID	r.m.s. fit	Z-score	%N	% SS equiv.
Elastase, 7EST(E)	Trypsin	β–Trypsin, 4PTP	Trypsin	—	35	1.2	9.5	68	100
T-cell surface glycoprotein, 3CD4(I)	Immunoglobulin	Bence-Jones dimer, 1REI(A)	Immunoglobulin	2,3,4,5	18	2.2	4.6	44	75
T-cell surface glycoprotein, 3CD4(II)	Immunoglobulin	T Lymphocyte antigen, CD2(I)	Immunoglobulin	4,6,7,11	15	4.1	3.9	11	83
Lactate dehydrogenase, 6LDH	Rossmann + catalytic 4MDH(A)	Malate dehydrogenase,	Rossmann + catalytic	2,3,4,5	15	2.6	4.5	52	71
Hexokinase B 2YHX,	Actin	1 1phh Nuc/bin Actin 2 1ATN(A) Actin		12	12	9.1	3.9	6	25

Chaperone protein, PapD(I)	Immunoglobulin	T-cell surface glycoprotein, 3CD4(I)	Immunoglobulin	3,9,15,16	10	4.5	5.3	37	57
Glycolate oxidase, 1GOX	αβ-Barrel 1WSY(A)	Trytophan synthase,	αβ-Barrel	6,29,30,36	10	13.8	1.8	32	63
D-xylose isomerase, 4XIA(A)	αβ-Barrel	Glycolate oxidase, 1GOX	αβ-Barrel	20,21,32,36	7	12.1	3.1	15	66
C-phycocyanin, 1CPC(B)	Globin	Myoglobin, 1MBA	Globin	2,3,5,13	7	7.4	3.8	34	57
Cytochrome B562,bundle 256b(A)	4-helix 2MHR	Myohemerythrin, bundle	4-helix	—	6	3.9	1.7	0	50

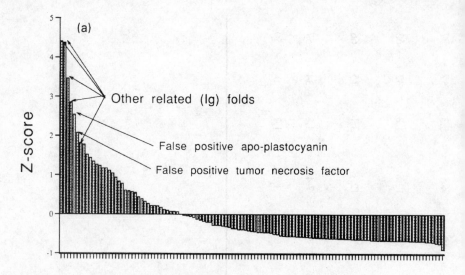

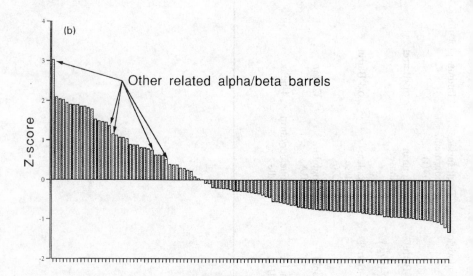

Fig. 3 Profiles of the Z-score for fold recognition. (a) The first domain of CD4 that identified immunoglobulin (Ig) folds at the first, second, third and fourth best matches. (b) Xylose isomerase showing matches of other $(\alpha\beta)8$ barrels.

contour map. A soft potential is used to check each possible pair of maps for surface complementarity. The second filter was to ensure there was a large area of interactions between the two protein surfaces. The third filter removed docked arrangements with unfavourable charge/charge interactions, which was evaluated by a simplified model for the side chains that was sufficiently soft to allow for some side chain movement on docking from the unbound structures. This approach always found a structure close to the crystallographic arrangement. At the interface the r.m.s. deviation for Ca atoms ranged from 1.9 to 3.4 Å for the 3 crystallographic structures and 4.7 Å when the predicted D1.3 structure was used (coordinates supplied by Drs Chothia and Lesk) to dock into the complex.

The problem was that several equally favourable alternatives were identified. Typically this number of alternatives was in the hundreds. At the same time several other groups were developing and applying protein/protein docking algorithms and were obtaining similar results. The key problem was one of selecting the correctly docked structure from a series of alternate, seemingly equally favourable arrangements.

To tackle the screening problem we have re-examined some of the potential energy terms used to evaluate the favourability of protein/protein interactions. The energy function uses a continuum model to estimate the hydrophobic free energy and electrostatic effects.

Most models for the hydrophobic free energy were based on the experimental free energy of transfer of non-polar residues from water to a non-polar solvent being modelled by an empirical proportionality to the change in solvent accessible area (20–30 cal mol^{-1} Å^{-2} of *accessible* surface). However recently Honig and co-workers (Sharp *et al.*, 1991), proposed that the experimental free energy changes need to be corrected for the differing sizes of the solutes and solvent. They also introduced a second correction based on the curvature of the surface to reconcile the difference between macroscopic surface tension and its microscopic manifestation (the hydrophobic effect). This effectively doubled the hydrophobic effect (to 46 cal mol^{-1} Å^{-2} of *accessible* surface). It was suggested that this increased value was in agreement with the experimental results of deleting methylene groups in point mutations.

We have applied scaled particle theory (Pierotti, 1976) to model the hydrophobic effect (Jackson and Sternberg, 1993, 1994). The formation of a solution is modelled as a two state process—first the progressive scaling up of the formation of a cavity in the solvent, followed by the introduction of the solute into the cavity. The study showed that transfer data and the effects of hydrophobic point mutations can be rationalized without the need to introduce a correction for the differing sizes of solute and solvent. The hydrophobic effect could be modelled by a proportionality to the change in molecular surface (69 cal mol^{-1} Å^{-2} of *molecular* surface). In contrast to a model based on accessible area, the relationship of the hydrophobic effect with molecular surface could be extended to surfaces of varied curvature and to model interactions ranging from the dimerization of methane to protein–protein docking. Thus we used the change in molecular surface to model the hydrophobic effect of docking.

Electrostatic effects are estimated by finite difference solutions to the Poisson–Boltzmann equation implemented in the program DelPhi (Gilson and Honig, 1988). This method calculates electrostatic potentials for molecules of arbitrary shapes and charge distributions. Different dielectrics can be assigned to the protein and the solvent. Two electrostatic effects are modelled. First there is the unfavourable desolvation on binding, and then the, potentially favourable, electrostatic interaction.

Previously, Shoichet and Kuntz (1991) generated a set of proteinase/inhibitor complexes using their DOCK algorithm but were unable to identify the correct answer despite the use of a series of different functions. We applied our continuum model to their generated complexes (Jackson and Sternberg, 1995). On the three bound and corresponding three unbound proteinase/inhibitor complexes, our potential function identified the near native complex from the alternative false dockings (Fig. 3). The r.m.s. Cα differences between the predicted and best possible docking ranged from 0.71 to 1.93 Å for the unbound complexes (Fig. 4 and Plate 2).

The success of our screening encouraged us to tackle the docking challenge. Professor James issued the three-dimensional coordinates of β-lactamase and its inhibitor and challenged the theoretical community to predict the docked conformation. To maintain consistency with our work on screening, we started by obtaining from Drs Shoichet and Kuntz a set of complexes generated by their DOCK algorithm. We then screened this series of complexes and identified a single structure that was our best prediction, guided mainly by the estimated energy of the interaction. After submission, our prediction was found to be 2.1 Å away from the correct conformation. Other groups in the world tackled the problem. Some obtained similar results but had less confidence in their screening, submitting series of dock structures. Other groups failed to find the correct answer.

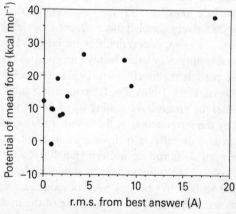

Fig. 4 Screening the predicted complexes of chymotrypsin and ovomucoid. The component proteins were docked in their unbound conformations using DOCK (Shoichet and Kuntz, 1991). For each complex the potential of mean force (in kcal mol^{-1}) is plotted against the r.m.s. deviation in Å for Cα atoms between the complex and the best possible prediction (i.e. 0.0 r.m.s. deviation obtained by superposing the unbound components on the bound coordinates).

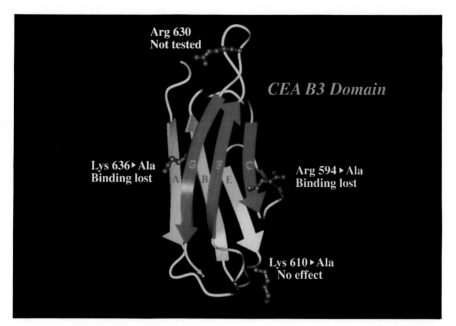

Plate 1a The predicted three-dimensional structure of the membrane-proximal domain of carcinoembrionic antigen (CEA). The roles of four putative residues that might be in the PR1A3 epitope were probed by mutagenesis.

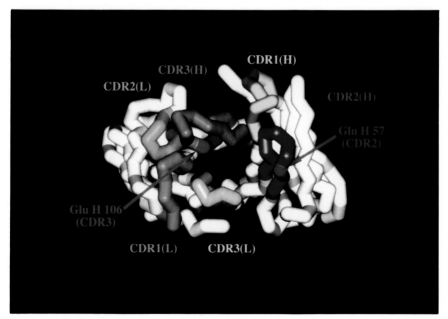

Plate 1b The predicted three-dimensional structure of monoclonal PR1A3 showing the location of two glutamic acid residues in the combining site.

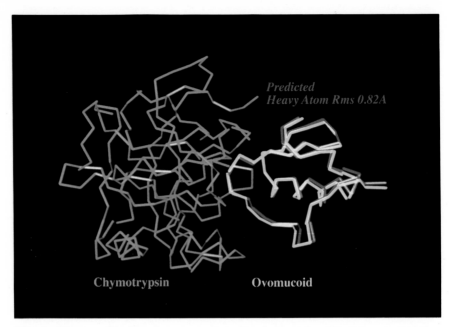

Plate 2 Diagram of the lowest energy conformation (magenta) and the 0.0 r.m.s. deviation conformation (yellow) for the predicted complexes of chymotrypsin and ovomucoid based on DOCK (see Chapter 5, Fig. 4).

Our work on DAPMATCH and the continuum screening of the results from DOCK are based on rigid body docking. Clearly the next step is to extend this approach to include conformational flexibility, initially of side chains.

5 Conclusion

The last few years has shown that there has been substantial progress in protein modelling. The possibility of identifying that a new sequence will thread onto a known fold provides promise that structure predictions can be extended beyond obvious homologies. However both for homology building and fold recognition, the challenge remains one of obtaining the correct sequence alignments. The results of the docking challenge, albeit on one system, suggest that the structures of complexes might be predicted from knowledge of the component structures when there is little conformational change on docking. These developments, together with the increase in the number of experimentally determined protein structures, will markedly extend the range of protein targets for which structural information can be obtained computationally.

References

Bairoch, A. and Boeckmann, B. (1991). *Nucl. Acid Res.* **19**, 2247–2249.
Barton, G. J. and Sternberg, M. J. E. (1987). *Prot. Eng.* **1**, 89–94.
Bates, P. A. and Sternberg, M. J. E. (1992). In *Protein Engineering—A Practical Approach,* (A. R. Rees, M. J. E. Sternberg and R. Wetzel, eds), pp. 117–141. Oxford University Press, Oxford.
Bates, P. A., Luo, J. and Sternberg, M. J. E. (1992). *FEBS Letts.* **301**, 207–214.
Bernstein, F. C., Koetzle, T. F., Williams, G., Meyer, D. J., Brice, M. D., Rodgers, J. R., Kennard, O., Shimanouchi, T. and Tasumi, M. (1977). *J. Mol. Biol.* **112**, 535–542.
Blundell, T. L., Sibanda, B. L., Sternberg, M. J. E. and Thornton, J. M. (1987). *Nature* **326**, 347–352.
Bowie, J. U., Lüthy, R. and Eisenberg, D. (1991). *Science* **253**, 164–170.
Chothia, C., Lesk, A. M., Tramontano, A., Levitt, M., Smith, G. S., Air, G., Sheriff, S., Padlan, E. A., Davies, D., Tulip, W. R., Colman, P. M., Spinelli, S., Alzari, P. M. and Poljak, R. J. (1989). *Nature (Lond.)* **342**, 877–883.
Dayhoff, M. (1978). *Atlas of Protein Sequence and Structure.* National Biomedical Research Foundation, Silver Spring, MD.
Gilson, M. K. and Honig, B. (1988). *Prot. Struct Funct. Genet.* **4**, 7–18.
Jackson, R. M. and Sternberg, M. J. E. (1993). *Nature* **366**, 638.
Jackson, R. M. and Sternberg, M. J. E. (1994). *Prot. Eng.* **7**, 371–383.
Jackson, R. M. and Sternberg, M. J. E. (1995). *J. Mol. Biol.* **250**, 258–275.
Jones, D. T., Taylor, W. R. and Thornton, J. M. (1992). *Nature* **358**, 86–89.
Jones, T. A. and Thirup, S. (1986). *EMBO J.* **5**, 819–822.
Martin, A. C. R., Cheetham, J. C. and Rees, A. R. (1989). *Proc. Natl. Acad. Sci., USA* **86**, 9268–9272.
Nishikawa, K. and Ooi, T. (1980). *Int. J. Peptide Protein Res.* **16**, 19–32.
Orengo, C. A., Jones, D. T. and Thornton, J. M. (1994). *Nature* **372**, 631–634.
Perutz, M. F. (1992). *Protein Structure: New Approaches to Disease and Therapy.* W. H. Freeman, San Francisco.

Pierotti, R. A. (1976). *Chem. Rev.* **76**, 717–726.
Rost, B. and Sander, C. (1993). *J. Mol. Biol.* **232**, 584–599.
Sharp, K. A., Nicholls, A., Fine, R. F. and Honig, B. (1991). *Science* **252**, 106–109.
Shoichet, B. K. and Kuntz, I. D. (1991). *J. Mol. Biol.* **221**, 327–346.
Shortle, D. (1995). *Nature Struct. Biol.* **2**, 91–93.
Walls, P. H. and Sternberg, M. J. E. (1992). *J. Mol. Biol.* **228**, 277–297.

III

FROM GENE TO TARGET

6

Expressing the Unknown: Considerations in Heterologous Expression of Novel Gene Products to Optimize Determination of their Functions

ALLAN R. SHATZMAN

SmithKline Beecham Pharmaceuticals, King of Prussia, PA 19406–2799, USA

Abstract

The focus of much of the literature on heterologous gene expression over the last 10–15 years has been on efforts to achieve very high levels of expression. One typically bowed his or her head in shame unless expression levels of $g\,l^{-1}$ could be reached and tears flowed like a river if a cell did not swell with the recombinant protein of interest, reaching levels of 30–50% of total cell protein. The fact that these proteins were often improperly processed or insoluble was at most a minor annoyance. I cannot help but feel that such concerns have become almost meaningless when the subject of heterologous gene expression is focused on the expression of genes of unknown function. If we are to make sense out of the information which is being harvested from the human genome, the focus must be on product quality rather than quantity.

As one searches the various databases which house the growing information on the human genome, attention is rapidly drawn to those putative coding sequences with homology to known proteins of potential interest. Great care must be taken not to confuse the term homology with identity. Therefore, the first rule in expressing the unknown is to remember that the gene you are working with is indeed of unknown function. Do not assume that you know what the function of the protein will be once you have expressed it. Something that looks like a dopamine receptor may indeed encode a seven transmembrane receptor, but it may wind up being a novel serotonin receptor. A human gene which has 40% homology to a yeast transcription factor may have nothing to do with transcription at all in human beings! Do not even assume that you know whether or not the gene encodes a secreted product or that you can correctly predict what the authentic N-terminus is supposed to be if it is indeed a secreted gene product. If you produce the protein in an insoluble form, can you ever be completely sure that you have refolded it properly? If the gene product is expressed as a fusion protein, is the fusion partner likely to interfere with activity? Is the gene product supposed to be processed post-translationally and, if so, is that post-translational processing crucial to activity? How can a balance be achieved between assuring product quality/authenticity and getting some functional data quickly to know if the gene is really encoding something worth spending your time working on?

While there are no clear-cut answers to these questions, there *are* clear strategies which can be put in place when embarking on the journey to express the unknown. These strategies, some of which will be discussed in this chapter, can improve your chances (but never guarantee them) to solve the mystery and assign a function to a previously unknown gene product: and just think, there are 50 000–100 000 of these mysteries waiting to be solved.

1 Introduction

The 'engineering' of living organisms to alter their genetic make up has taken place since the beginning of time (see Fig. 1): only back then it was called 'survival of the fittest' or 'natural selection'. Those organisms whose altered patterns of gene expression provided them with an advantage which afforded survival passed on that genetic information to the following generations. One only need to look at a phylogenetic tree to comprehend how such naturally occurring changes in gene expression have led to the diversity of life that is evident today. During the last several hundred years (at least), humans have intervened in this process of altering the patterns of gene expression in living systems. The era of modern genetics was born in the early 1800s with the basic understanding of genetics which allowed one to choose those organisms which had a particular naturally occurring trait and intentionally breed them to give rise to an entire generation with that particular trait (e.g. flower colour). In the 1920s (about 100 years later) came the understanding that one could increase the rate of mutations (e.g. by use of X-rays or other radiation sources, or by adding chemical mutagens) and then select desired characteristics. This methodology is still used today (e.g. mutagenesis of the antibiotic-producing bacteria) to bring about genetic diversity and along with it, new forms of life-saving medicines. From that point forward, our understanding of how we can alter patterns in gene expression has grown exponentially. In early applications of what we today commonly refer to as 'molecular biology,' scientists used genetic manipulations to select *in vivo* recombination events which resulted in the introduction or deletion of particular genes into microorganisms. Today, through the uses of plasmids, phages and viruses, we are able to direct the synthesis of virtually any gene product in simple and complex organisms alike; and we can usually do it in a matter of days or weeks!

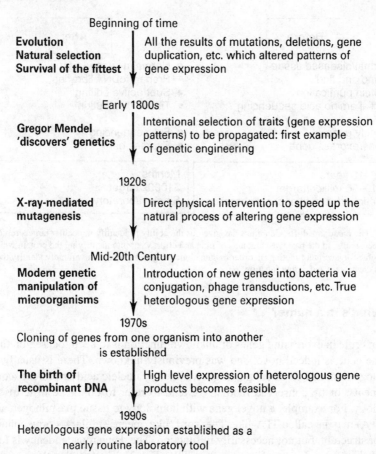

Beginning of time

Evolution
Natural selection
Survival of the fittest

All the results of mutations, deletions, gene duplication, etc. which altered patterns of gene expression

Early 1800s

Gregor Mendel
'discovers' genetics

Intentional selection of traits (gene expression patterns) to be propagated: first example of genetic engineering

1920s

X-ray-mediated
mutagenesis

Direct physical intervention to speed up the natural process of altering gene expression

Mid-20th Century

Modern genetic
manipulation of
microorganisms

Introduction of new genes into bacteria via conjugation, phage transductions, etc. True heterologous gene expression

1970s
Cloning of genes from one organism into another
is established

The birth of
recombinant DNA

High level expression of heterologous gene products becomes feasible

1990s
Heterologous gene expression established as a
nearly routine laboratory tool

Fig. 1 The genetic engineering time line. A brief look at this time line reveals that altering the expression patterns in living organisms is not really something new. It is the speed and precision with which we can now accomplish these changes that has revolutionized the field of genetics and created the field of biotechnology.

Despite these technological advances, the expression of recombinant gene products remains an art form where each gene must be considered on a case-by-case basis. The steps needed to produce any given protein in a functional manner are not always predictable and can vary drastically, even among genes which encode proteins closely related in structure and function. This problem is exacerbated by the fact that in this era of genomics, the paradigm by which genes are studied has been reversed. In the past, we have sought out genes which encoded proteins which were first identified through identification of their function. We now have genes which we must transform into proteins in order to identify their functions (Fig. 2). We must therefore focus our attention on not only achieving expression of the desired gene product, but on doing it in a way that is most likely to produce the protein in its native form; without the 'luxury' of knowing what that form may be!

Before	After
• Normal/diseased tissue • 'Grind and find' • Protein purification • Partial amino acid sequencing • Identify gene • Clone/express gene	• Normal/diseased tissue • Prepare cDNA libraries • Subtractive editing • Tissue distribution • Full sequencing • Express gene
• 10–15 years • $10–50 million/target • National/international collaboration	Months $1000s/target Single laboratory

Fig. 2 The paradigm shift. Genomics has given us the ability to identify molecular targets rapidly and less expensively. In the past, vast amounts of time and effort went into identifying the protein which was responsible for a certain function (in order to then clone the gene). We can now rapidly identify the gene, express the protein and define function.

2   What's in a name?

The first rule in expressing genes of unknown function is to keep focused on the fact that the gene is indeed novel and was previously unknown. There is usually some homology assigned to an unknown gene, either by nucleic acid or protein sequence alignments, or by conserved motifs. We tend to refer to this gene in terms of its homology. For example, a novel gene with homology to tissue plasminogen activator (TPA) may be called TPA-like. The word 'like' means similar—corresponding in type or structure, but not necessarily in function. The dangerous tendency is to drop the 'like' suffix and start referring to it as TPA (Fig. 3). The fact that this novel gene may encode a protein with a kringle or protease domain (thus making it TPA-like) does not make it TPA. That is not to say that the homology data is not very important in helping one decide how to express the novel gene product, and perhaps what type of assays to try first in order to assign function. If there is considerable literature describing what systems have worked well (and what have not) for expressing the known homologue in an active form (without *in vitro* manipulations such as refolding), it is reasonable to expect that the novel gene *may* behave similarly. Expression of gene products tends to be somewhat reproducible when the structures are well conserved as opposed to being dependent on conservation of amino acid sequence (e.g. many different sequences can yield similar structures).

2.1   Detecting expression of unknown gene products

Prior to expressing a gene which encodes a protein of unknown function, a plan must be in place for how you are going to detect expression. There are two primary approaches which are commonly used to address this issue (Fig. 4). The first

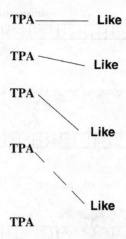

Fig. 3 The disappearing simile. One of the easiest traps to fall into is to start thinking of the gene of unknown function as encoding the protein to which homology has been assigned. It does not take more than one or two amino acid changes to alter the function of an enzyme or receptor. If thinking is restricted by the name that comes up on a homology search, you will miss all but the obvious.

approach involves generation of a polyclonal antisera without ever having purified any of the novel gene product. This may be accomplished by synthesizing several peptides from different regions encoded by the gene, and using these peptides to immunize small animals (e.g. mice or rabbits). Computer algorithms exist which can help to predict which peptides are most likely to represent regions of the protein which are expected to be surface exposed and therefore most likely to lead to anti-sera which will recognize the native, folded protein. Alternatively, immune responses to the protein of interest may be generated by direct injection of DNA into animals using non-replicating DNA expression vectors (Montgomery *et al.*, 1994). In this approach, the coding sequence for the gene is inserted downstream from a strong mammalian promoter (e.g. the promoter and enhancer form the cytomegalovirus immediate early gene 1) on a plasmid vector. This plasmid DNA is then injected into the animal (typically intramuscularly) where production of the protein peaks after about 7 days, and is maintained for many weeks, if not months (Wolff *et al.*, 1992; Manthorpe *et al.*, 1993). High titre antisera have been obtained by this method for a growing number of antigens including HIV-GP160 (Wang *et al.*, 1993; Nabel *et al.*, 1993), influenza virus NP (Ulmer *et al.*, 1993) and human growth hormone (Tang *et al.*, 1992). A third method of generating a specific antisera which is likely to recognize the native protein involves the use of live recombinant viral vectors (which have been engineered to express the protein of interest) to infect animals which in turn will produce the desired immune response (Mahr and Payne, 1992; Graham and Prevec, 1992).

The second approach to detecting expression of novel gene products is the addition of a peptide tag to the protein during systhesis (Fig. 4). This tag can not only serve

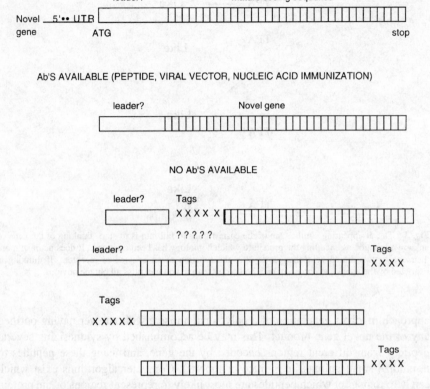

Fig. 4 Detection of novel gene expression. When working with a novel gene, a lot of guesswork may be involved, leading to a lot of room for errors. You often are left guessing how to trim the 5′ UTR. Is there a signal sequence and, if so, where does the mature protein start? These issues make designing expression strategies difficult. To complicate the matter, a strategy must be developed for detection of the unknown gene product. One can raise polyclonal antisera against the gene product by expressing the gene directly in an animal through the use of viral vectors or nucleic acid immunization. Alternatively, one can raise antisera against peptides derived from the translation of the coding sequence. If the above strategies are not viable, tags may be added on to the N or C terminal ends of the coding sequence. These tags can facilitate detection and purification. This approach is straightforward for non-secreted proteins but difficult for secreted products as it is nothing but guesswork if you wish to have the protein secreted with an N-terminal tag.

to facilitate detection, but can also be used in a generic purification step to isolate novel proteins for which no information exists to design more classical purification schemes. There are two main systems commonly used for tagging recombinant proteins, a polyhistidine tail or a linear epitope recognized by a monoclonal antibody.

A stretch of histidines (six tandem histidine residues being most common) can be added to either the N or C terminus of novel gene products using common molecular biological methods such as polymerase chain reaction (PCR). Addition of six histidine residues to the protein adds only 0.72 kDa to the mass of the protein, whereas other fusion protein systems typically utilize much larger affinity groups that must often be removed to allow normal protein function (note: these fusion protein systems will be discussed later on in the *Escherichia coli* expression section). The small histidine tail is not immunogenic and therefore need not be removed before the protein is used for immunization of animals to generate antisera. Histidine tailed proteins often retain their normal biological functions (e.g. dihydrofolate reductase and adenylate cyclase (Hochuli *et al.*, 1988; Taussig *et al.*, 1993)). The expression of a histidine-tagged protein can be readily detected using a modification of the Western blotting technique (O'Shannessy, personal communication). The cell lysate or media which contains the protein of interest is subjected to SDS PAGE with subsequent transfer of the proteins to nitrocellulose. In place of an antibody solution, the nitrocellulose is exposed to a nickel-chelate resin which has been conjugated with biotin. This resin binds with very high affinity to the hexahistidine tail as opposed to the cellular proteins which do not typically contain such a polyhistidine stretch. The biotinylated reagent may then be visualized using many of the commercially available reagents used in Western blotting (e.g. streptavidin conjugated horse radish peroxidase). The affinity of histidine residues for immobilized Ni^{2+} ions also allows selective purification of these tagged proteins from very complex mixtures (e.g. whole cell lysates or fermentation broths). This high affinity (K_d of 10^{-13}) permits purification steps to be conducted in the presence of detergents or chaotropic agents such as urea and guanidine (Hochuli *et al.*, 1988; Stuber *et al.*, 1990). The protein can be easily eluted from this resin using imidazole buffers.

The second commonly used protein tagging system employs a linear peptide epitope for which a high affinity monoclonal antibody exists. This peptide is fused to the protein of interest using the same methods one would employ for attaching a polyhistidine tail. The monoclonal antibody can then be used to detect expression using a traditional Western blotting method, and can also be used to generate an affinity column to purify the protein of interest. One common peptide tag is the Flag peptide (Hopp *et al.*, 1988) which encodes an eight amino acid-long sequence (DYKDDDDK). The first four amino acids of this tag provide the epitope for the high affinity monoclonal antibody while the C-terminal portion encodes an enterokinase cleavage site for removal of the tag from the purified protein. An alternative to the Flag peptide is the haemagglutinin peptide tag system (Pati, 1992). This system employs the peptide sequence YPYDVPDYA and the high affinity monoclonal antibody 12CA5 which is specific for this epitope.

The histidine tag and epitope tag methods, while each powerful in their own right, have certain limitations. Detection of epitope-tagged proteins with a highly specific monoclonal antibody gives somewhat cleaner results than the histidine-tagged system. The ability to purify rapidly the epitope-tagged proteins produced using virtually any expression system is far more predictable when using a monoclonal antibody affinity column when compared to purification using metal chelate chromatography. While a monoclonal antibody is typically very specific, many histidine-rich proteins will be recognized by nickel resin (with differing affinities) leading to high backgrounds. In addition, many media formulations contain components which can interfere with metal chelate chromatography and make purification of secreted proteins difficult. Nickel chelate, however, is far superior to monoclonal antibody purification procedures with regard to flexibility (purification can be done in the presence of detergents and denaturants), and very small columns can be used to purify relatively large amounts of protein. In order to obtain the greatest sensitivity and flexibility in detecting and purifying the unknown, it may therefore be advisable to add both tags to the end of the novel gene product.

2.2 Is there an end in sight?

The next consideration in expressing the unknown is designing the insertion of the coding sequence into the expression vector. It may sometimes be difficult, if not impossible, to predict where the N-terminal end of the protein is supposed to be. A signal sequence does not always look like a signal sequence, and when it does, you cannot always predict where the native signal sequence cleavage site should be. There is at least one case I can recall where a gene of unknown function was expressed using the native N-terminal coding sequence which may or may not have encoded a signal sequence. The gene was expressed in two different eukaryotic expression systems; in one system it was secreted while in the other it remained cytoplasmic! With this level of unpredictability, it is best to leave the 5' end of the coding sequence alone and let nature try to tell you what is right and what is not, and if you must modify the coding sequence (e.g. add a tag for detection purposes), add it to the 3' end—at least we think we know where the stop codon is!

2.3 Expressing the unknown—E. coli

Escherichia coli is the most commonly used system for expression of heterologous gene products. This is due, at least in part, to the short time frame needed to develop an expressing strain, the high levels of expression one can expect, and the relatively simple recombinant DNA techniques necessary to work with this system (Fig. 5a). The vast knowledge of *E. coli* genetics and physiology which has been accumulated over the last 20–30 years is an equally important factor in making *E. coli* the 'work horse' of the gene expression field. For all of its advantages, *E. coli* has some very major disadvantages as well. Many eukaryotic proteins, when expressed in *E. coli,* do not fold properly and often precipitate within the cell in insoluble aggregates referred to as inclusion bodies. Secondly, eukaryotic proteins produced in *E. coli* are not properly modified at the post-transcriptional level (e.g. glycosylation). Finally, *E. coli* is not amenable to high level secretion of proteins into the surrounding media, with most exported proteins being localized in the periplasmic space which separates the inner and outer cell membranes. This of course is compounded by the fact that the mammalian leader sequence on the novel gene needs to be removed (when you do not even know if there is one or where it ends) and to be replaced by an *E. coli* leader sequence to get the protein into the periplasm. Despite all of these negatives, many will insist on expressing genes of unknown function in *E. coli* because of its technical ease. Described below are some strategies which may help to achieve success.

(a)

Pros

● Easy
● Fast
● High yields

Cons

● Improper folding
● Insolubility
● Lack of appropriate post-translational modification
● Need to predict authentic N-terminal of novel gene product
● *In vitro* refolding is not quantifiable—do not know what native structure or function is!

(b)

■ **Slow the rate of expression**
  – lower concentration of inducing agent
  – lower growth/induction temperature

■ **Co-expression of chaperone proteins**

■ **Secretion**

■ **Protein fusions**

Fig. 5 (a) Pros and cons associated with expressing genes of unknown function in *E. coli*. (b) Strategies for expressing genes of unknown function in *E. coli* to optimize chances for functionality.

2.4 What's wrong with E. coli and what can you do about it?

Among the most common problems encountered with expression of heterologous gene products in *E. coli* is improper protein folding which may lead to aggregation and the formation of insoluble inclusion bodies. While there are, at present, no panaceas to this problem, there are several approaches which have been shown to be helpful in particular cases (Fig. 5b). Slowing the rate of expression can help improve solubility of some proteins (Mizukani *et al.*, 1986). This can be achieved in a number of ways, such as lowering the concentration of inducing agent (e.g. IPTG) or lowering the copy number of the plasmid used to direct the gene of interest. Lowering the temperature at which the protein is being produced can similarly result in improved solubility as many proteins are more soluble at lower temperatures (Schein, 1989). Lower temperatures also can help to slow the kinetics of synthesis, thus providing a double benefit. There is also an increasing body of evidence which suggests that co-expression of specialized proteins called 'chaperones' can aid in the folding process and result in improved solubility for a number of gene products (Gilbert, 1994). Finally, proteins which are often insoluble when produced intracellularly are found to be soluble when secreted into the periplasmic space or extracellular media. While *E. coli* is not particularly well suited for secreting large amounts of protein, recent advances in *E. coli* secretion systems have made this a viable alternative.

Expression of a gene product in an authentic or nearly authentic form is often most desirable as it favours correct structure and function. Expression of an authentic gene product is often quite difficult and time consuming. Evaluating different transcription systems, altering codon content and A + T content, and varying production conditions can take months of effort with no guarantee of success. It is often quicker to solve expression-related problems by making fusions between genes. Gene fusions are typically constructed by fusing the gene of interest to the 5' end of a gene which has been proven to express at high levels in *E. coli*. While this fusion partner or carrier sequence is often from an *E. coli* gene, it can be from any well-expressed gene. The fusion partner can also consist of an entire gene or only a small portion of one. In addition to helping improve expression levels, the fusion partner may often provide an added benefit such as easing protein purification or improving heat stability. Protein fusions are most commonly used as a source of antigen for producing antibodies and, in many cases, can be used for biochemical analysis. Protein fusions also have some major drawbacks. Most importantly, production of a protein as a fusion may have dramatic negative effects on its activity and structure. The very high levels of expression one typically obtains with a fusion approach also tend to lead to the formation of inclusion bodies.

In the sections below, I will describe two different fusion systems which are commonly used today.

3 Glutathione-S-transferase fusion proteins

Glutathione-S-transferase (GST) fusions are commonly made using the pGEX vector system (Smith *et al.*, 1986; Smith, 1993). Genes are typically fused to the 3' end of the GST coding sequence. GST was originally cloned from *Schistosoma japonicum* and encodes a protein of 26 kDa. One reason that this system has gained popularity is that most proteins produced as GST fusions remain soluble when expressed in *E. coli* (Smith and Corcoran, 1994). This is in contrast to the formation of insoluble aggregates typically obtained when expressing proteins as fusion with *lacZ*, trp E, lambda cII, etc. Since the protein is soluble, the harsh denaturing conditions typically required for solubilization of inclusion bodies are not necessary, increasing the probability that the gene product of interest may retain its functional activity and immunoreactivity. The GST portion of the fusion also provides an easy, one step purification procedure for virtually any GST fusion protein. The cell lysate containing the GST fusion is passed over a column consisting of glutathione immobilized on agarose beads. The fusion protein binds to this column while most host proteins flow through. The protein can then be eluted using free reduced glutathione at neutral pH. GST preparations are typically ≥90% pure after this simple procedure. The GST system works best for smaller proteins, with solubility becoming less predictable as the size of the fusion protein increases above 50 kDa (Smith, 1993).

4 Thioredoxin fusion proteins

Thioredoxin gene fusions are used for high level production of heterologous gene products as C-terminal fusions to the thioredoxin gene from *E. coli* (LaVallie *et al.*, 1993a). As with the GST system described above, this system is particularly useful for the production of soluble fusion proteins. In many instances, thioredoxin fusion proteins are correctly folded and display full biological activity. Thioredoxin imparts unusual thermal stability to its fusion partner and its cellular localization makes fusion protein susceptible to quantitative release from *E. coli* by osmotic shock (LaVallie *et al.*, 1993a,b). Both of these features can be used to enhance purification of thioredoxin fusion proteins. Thioredoxin itself has somewhat remarkable properties when overexpressed in *E. coli*. The protein (MW ~12 kDa) can be produced at levels approaching 40% of total cellular protein and remains completely soluble even when present at those levels (Holmgren, 1985). These properties have enabled the production of many eukaryotic gene products as soluble thioredoxin fusion at very high levels (5–20% of total cell protein), proteins which were completely insoluble when produced at even much lower levels as non-fusion proteins (McCoy and LaVallie, 1994).

5 Cleavage of fusion proteins

Expression systems which generate soluble fusion proteins have revitalized the use of *E. coli* for the production of a large variety of gene products which otherwise would have required the use of more complex higher eukaryotic expression technologies. As a result of this popularity, the ability to cleave the N-terminal fusion carrier protein from the C-terminal gene product of interest has become increasingly important. Once the N-terminal fusion partner (be it protein or tag) has done its job of increasing solubility, facilitating purification, or allowing rapid detection, it has in general outlived its usefulness. The separation of the protein from its fusion partner is generally achieved by proteolytic cleavage at a site which had been specifically engineered between the C terminus of the fusion partner and the N terminus of the gene product of interest. Among the most common proteases used are factor Xa which recognizes the sequence Ile-Glu/ASP-Gly-Arg and enterokinase which recognizes the sequence Asp-Asp-Asp-Asp-Lys. The choice of which protease to use depends to a large extent on the protein sequence of the gene of interest, as this sequence must be closely examined to assure that it does not contain sites which might be recognized by one of these proteins. This is not generally a problem as these two proteases are among the most specific of all known proteases. That is not to say that unwanted digestion of the protein of interest is not a (sometimes) significant problem with these methods despite the specificity of factor Xa and enterokinase. Most commercially available sources of these proteases are purified from natural sources and contain trace levels of other proteins including far less specific proteases (LaVallie *et al.*, 1993b). For example, trypsin and chymotrypsin are often present in enterokinase which is purified from bovine intestines. As recombinant sources become more widely available (and more affordable) in the future, these problems will diminish significantly.

5.1   Expressing the unknown in mammalian cells

At the far end of the spectrum from the humble prokaryote *E. coli* is the highly complex mammalian cell. While expression systems utilizing mammalian cells are most likely to produce a human gene product in its native form (including appropriate post-translational modification), there are a number of limitations which constrain their use in the initial attempts to express the unknown in order to define function. Transient expression systems typically allow you to evaluate production of the product of interest within 2–3 days of introduction of the expression vector whereas several weeks or months may be required for generation of a stable cell line. However, the transient system may only produce microgram or sub-microgram quantities of the protein, making purification, even using tag technology, very difficult. In addition, mammalian cells commonly used in transient transfections (e.g. COS, HeLa, HEK293) grow as attached cells in serum-containing media which may contain animal proteins (e.g. cytokines) that can interfere with many biological assays. Despite these limitations, transient mammalian expression systems can prove to be very powerful in rapidly evaluating the function of novel gene products when very sensitive functional assays can be applied. For example, these systems have proven especially useful when expressing novel gene products with homolgy to seven-transmembrane receptors where changes in adenylate cyclase activity or calcium fluxes can be measured in response to ligand binding to novel receptors.

Generation of mammalian cell lines stably expressing recombinant gene products is undoubtedly the best way to optimize both the chances of producing the gene product of unknown function in an active form and in useful amounts. However, the time required to generate and expand such cell lines can range from several weeks to several months. It is therefore suggested to use other, more rapid systems, to produce initial quantities of a protein to determine if it has a function or properties you are interested in studying, and then use stable mammalian systems to provide long-term supplies of the gene product to allow extensive characterization.

5.2   Is there a middle ground?

Thus far, I have described the use of two expression systems which can be used to express the unknown, each with its own substantial advantages and drawbacks. *E. coli* is easy and rapid to use but there is substantial concern over product quality.

Mammalian systems, while optimal in terms of product quality, may not produce sufficient product to afford purification (with transient systems) or may take long periods of time to generate stable cell lines which produce the gene product of interest. Is there a middle ground: a system which provides for rapid expression of proteins in quantities sufficient to support purification in a relatively brief time frame? The answer is insect cell culture systems.

6 Heterologous gene expression in insect cells

6.1 The baculovirus system

Baculoviruses have become among the most popular systems (perhaps second only to *E. coli*) for overproducing recombinant proteins. Several key elements have contributed to this popularity. The baculovirus system is a eukaryotic system (typically using *Spodoptera frugiperda* cells) which is capable of carrying out many of the protein modification and processing events typical of higher eukaryotic systems. The baculovirus system uses a helper-independent virus that can be propagated to high titres in insect cells which can be grown in suspension culture (O'Reilly *et al.*, 1992; King and Possee, 1992). Unlike *E. coli*, high level intracellular expression of heterologous gene products in the baculovirus system does not give rise to inclusion bodies. Rather, proteins typically remain soluble, are properly folded, and biologically active (O'Reilly *et al.*, 1992). Upon infection of insect cells with recombinant baculoviruses, host protein synthesis is greatly reduced, leading to high levels of production and increased ease of purification for the recombinant gene product (Luckow, 1993).

Baculoviruses are a large group of insect viruses that contain a circular double-stranded DNA genome ranging in size from 80 to 220 kb in length (Doenflen and Bohm, 1986). The *Autographa californica* nuclear polyhedrosis virus (AcNPV) is the most popular form of the virus for heterologous gene expression purposes. The baculovirus life cycle is divided into immediate early, early, late and very late phases. Viruses enter the host cell by adsorptive endocytosis and release their DNA upon entry into the nucleus followed by replication of the viral genome. Two forms of viral progeny are produced, extracellular viral particles during late phase (up until ~18 h post-infection) and intracellular polyhedron-derived virus particles during the very late phase (18–72 h post-infection). The intracellular viral particles are filled with the polyhedrin protein (29 kDa) of baculovirus. While this polyhedrin protein serves an important survival role for the virus in nature, it is not necessary for the survival and propagation of virus in insect cell culture in the laboratory (Murphy and Pirvnica-Worms, 1994).

The baculovirus expression system relies heavily on polyhedrin biology for its utility. The regulatory signals which govern polyhedron synthesis are especially strong and efficient as polyhedrin constitutes up to 50% of cell protein in the very late stage of the infection cycle (Doenflen and Bohm, 1986). Viruses lacking the polyhedron gene (e.g. recombinant viruses) can be easily distinguished from wild-type viruses by simple visual inspection for altered plaque morphology. The coding sequence for the gene to be expressed is typically inserted downstream of the polyhedron promoter present on a baculovirus transfer vector. This vector is then transfected along with wild-type viral DNA into insect cells. The foreign gene is inserted into the viral genome by a homologous recombination event such that it replaces the polyhedron gene. Recent advances in baculovirus technology using defective virus and plasmid complementation have increased the frequency of obtaining recombinant virus from 0.2% up to 85–99% (Kitts and Possee, 1993). Recombinant viruses are chosen upon visual selection (absence of polyhedron inclusion bodies) under a light microscope, and amplified to produce a high titre stock. This recombinant viral stock is then used to infect insect tissue culture cells to produce the gene of interest. Although technically more complex, some elements of this system are far simpler than E. coli or yeast. There is generally only one promoter needed for consideration (as opposed to a shopping list for E. coli or yeast) and no obvious need to optimize the translation initiation signal as with E. coli.

This expression system has been used to produce hundreds of mammalian gene products over the last several years. Several reviews which focus on proteins which have been produced in this system along with comparisons of their biological properties as compared to their native source have been written in the last few years (e.g. Luckow, 1991). In general, the results are excellent. Cell surface receptors, ion channels, growth factors, plasma proteins, proteases and regulatory proteins (to name a few) have all been made successfully in this system. Baculovirus-infected insect cells perform many of the post-translational modifications of higher eukaryotes including glycosylation, fatty acid acylation (e.g. myristoylation), amino terminal acetylation, carboxy terminal α-amidation, and phosphorylation. Intracellular proteins are usually targeted to the appropriate cellular location (e.g. nucleus or cytoplasm) while inclusion of a baculovirus signal sequence usually assures efficient secretion. While obviously a powerful expression system, there are several cautions to keep in mind. Insect cell glycosylation is quite different to mammalian cell glycosylation (e.g. less complex with no sialic acid) and thus has many of the same concerns noted for yeast glycosylation. Expression of a mammalian gene with its natural leader sequence may be quite inefficient, often requiring insertion of the mature coding sequence downstream of a baculovirus signal sequence. This need to re-engineer the secretion signal, however, is not as absolute as was the case with E. coli or yeast. Baculovirus genes also do not contain introns, so the use of cDNAs rather than genomic clones is highly recommended (although there are some reports that proper splicing of heterologous genes may be possible; Jeang et al., 1987). Unlike the systems described previously, one does not generate a stable recombinant cell line which can be used to produce the recombinant gene product on a continued basis. The baculovirus system is a lytic system requiring continual propagation and purification of virus followed by infection of cells each time you wish to produce the recombinant gene product. This can become quite labour intensive when used for large-scale production. Finally, the time it takes to go from cloned gene to protein is now typically weeks rather than days (as it was when we started out with E. coli).

These factors, however, are often inconsequential when one is able to obtain the desired gene product in this system while *E. coli* failed to produce the desired results!

7 Heterologous gene expression in *Drosophila*

Although not nearly as widely used as the baculovirus system, cultured *Drosophila melanogaster* cells have proven to be outstanding hosts for the expression of heterologous gene products. *Drosophila* Schneider line 2 (S2) cells have many of the advantages (Fig. 6) of *Spedoptera* cells, such as room temperature growth in suspension to a high cell density, ability to produce authentic proteins of eukaryotic, prokaryotic, or viral origin, and the ability to carry out complex post-translational processing. Unlike the baculovirus system, the *Drosophila* expression system requires no virus and is not a lytic system. Transfection of S2 cells produces stable cell lines which can be used for continuous production of a foreign gene. In addition, mammalian leader sequences are generally recognized with equal efficiency to *Drosophila* leader sequences, negating the need to re-engineer signal sequences (Ivey-Hoyle, 1991).

Heterologous gene expression is generally obtained by cloning the gene of interest downstream of a strong, regulatable promoter. The *Drosophila* metallothionein promoter has been shown to produce high levels of protein in stably transfected S2 cells (Johansen *et al.*, 1989; Culp *et al.*, 1991). This promoter allows tightly regulated expression, even at very high copy number. Induction is accomplished simply by the addition of copper, analogous to the case described for IPTG inductions in *E. coli* or CUP induction in yeast.

The plasmid containing the gene of interest (cloned adjacent to the metallothionein promoter) is generally introduced into S2 cells by standard calcium phosphate transfection. A second plasmid encoding a selectable marker (resistance to

■ **S2 cells**
  – growth at room temperature
  – inexpensive serum-free media
  – suspension culture
  – high cell density (10^7 cells ml^{-1})

■ **Stable expression**
  – constitutive and inducible promoters
  – up to 1000 gene copies/cell without amplification
  – stability for 60+ passages

■ **Transient expression**

Fig. 6 Advantages of the *Drosophila* expression system. The ability to culture S2 cells in suspension in serum-free media provides a distinct advantage over many higher eukaryotic cell lines. High levels of expression when used in either transient or stable expression make this system among the most versatile.

G418 or hygromycin) is co-transfected in order to select for stable cell lines. Within about 3 weeks, stable cell lines carrying the two vector sequences integrated into the chromosome in a multi-copy tandem array are obtained. Copy numbers as high as 1000/cell have been obtained for some heterologous genes introduced into S2 cells in this way (Johansen *et al.*, 1989). In general, expression levels increase with increasing copy number, though the increase is non-linear as one reaches very high gene copy number. This ability to establish rapidly stable cell lines without the need for time-consuming amplification steps has enabled us to develop S2 cell lines expressing from 50 000 (endothelin receptor) to 250 000 (IL-5 receptor) receptors/ cell (Fig. 7). The system can also be used for co-expressing several proteins simultaneously, simply by adding additional vectors into the transfection process. By varying the relative amounts of each plasmid, you can vary the relative expression level of each gene product. Co-expression of antibody heavy and light chain genes has been demonstrated to yield monoclonal antibodies that are equivalent in affinity to the identical monoclonal antibody produced in mammalian systems. Even more complex functional $GABA_A$ receptors which form pentameric structures composed of three different subunits have been successfully expressed in this system. Typical expression levels for secreted gene products (e.g. cytokines and soluble receptors) are in the 10–50 mg l^{-1} range following a 7 day induction period of a stable cell line, while expression of viral antigens (e.g. HIV GP120 and RSV F protein) is typically in the 1–5 mg l^{-1} range. As noted for the baculovirus system, virtually any type of protein can be produced in a soluble, active, and properly folded form using the *Drosophila* system. Seven-transmembrane receptors, cytokines, and even antibodies have been routinely produced using S2 cells (Kirkpatrick *et al.*, in preparation). *Drosophila* S2 cells can also be transiently transfected producing 1–5 mg l^{-1} of many desired gene products in as little as 3 days.

- **Secreted proteins**
  - cytokines/cytokine receptors
  - mAbs
  - viral antigens

- **Lethal gene products**

- **Cell-based assays**

- **Expression of complex receptors**
  - single transmembrane
  - seven transmembrane
  - ion channels

Fig. 7 Applications of the *Drosophila* expression system. We have used this system to express successfully virtually every kind of gene product. S2 cells can support expression of complex receptor molecules, secreted proteins, intracellular enzymes and transcription factors. The lack of many mammalian homologues makes this system ideal for the development of cell-based assays with virtually no background.

8 Concluding remarks

No one system can ever be expected to express every gene product in a functional form. One must carefully select a group of systems which is best suited to the class of protein(s) which is under investigation. The type of assays to be used to detect function must be considered prior to choosing an expression system as cellular backgrounds vary drastically (e.g. CHO cells have a high basal calcium flux whereas HEK293 cells do not). Insect cells are quite suitable for evaluating expression of novel receptors when using radiolabelled ligands, but perhaps not when looking for signal transduction. One must always remember that the function to be defined in an *in vitro* assay or even in an animal model may have nothing to do with the actual function of that protein in the human body. One must also remember that human cell types can vary greatly with respect to the types of genes that they express and the types of post-translational modifications they carry out. A human kidney cell line may not replicate identically the modifications which take place when the same protein is produced in a human T-cell. With these caveats in mind, we should still expect to be successful in defining the functions of virtually every gene which is expressed in the human genome, leaving us with the puzzle of how these 50–100 000 activities come together to orchestrate the functioning human body.

References

Culp, J. S., Johansen, H., Hellmig, B., Beck, J., Matthews, T. J., Delers, A. and Rosenberg, M. (1991). *Biotechnology* **9**, 173–178.
Doenflen, W. and Bohm, P. (1986). In *The Molecular Biology of Baculoviruses*. Springer-Verlag, New York.
Gilbert, H. F. (1994). *Curr. Opin. Biotechnol.* **5**, 534–539.
Graham, F. L. and Prevec, L. (1992). *Biotechnology* **20**, 363–390.
Hochuli, E., Bannwarth, W., Dobeli, H., Genyz, R. and Stuber, D. (1988). *Bio/Technology* **6**, 1321–1325.
Holmgren, A. (1985). *Annu. Rev. Biochem.* **54**, 237–271.
Hopp, T. P., Prickett, K. S., Price, V. L., Libby, R. T., March, C. J., et. al. (1988). *Bio/Technology* **6**, 1204–1210.
Ivey-Hoyle, M. (1991). *Curr. Opin. Biotechnol.* **2**, 704–707.
Jeang, K., Giam, C., Nerenberg, M. and Khoury, G. (1987). *J. Virol.* **61**, 708–713.
Johansen, H., Van Der Straten, A., Sweet, R., Otto, E., Maroni, G. and Rosenberg, M. (1989) *Gene Devel.* **3**, 173–178.
King, L. A. and Possee, R. D. (1992). In *The Baculovirus Expression System: A Laboratory Guide*, pp. 1–229. Chapman and Hall, London.
Kirkpatrick, R. et al., In preparation.
Kitts, P. A. and Possee, R. D. (1993). *Bio Techniques* **14**, 810–817.
LaVallie, E. R., DiBlasio, E. A., Kovacic, S., Grant, K. L., Schendel, P. F. and McCoy, J. M. (1993a). *Bio/Technology* **11**, 187–193.
LaVallie, E. R., Rehemtulla, A., Racie, L. A., DiBlasio, E. A. Ferenz, C. Grant, K. L., Light, A. and McCoy, J. M. (1993b). *J. Biol. Chem.* **268**, 23311-23317.
Luckow, V. A. (1991). In *Recombinant DNA Technology and Applications* (A. Prokop, R. K. Bojpal and C. Ho, eds), pp. 97–152. McGraw Hill, New York.

Luckow, V. A. (1993). *Curr. Opin. Biotechnol.* **4**, 564–572.

Mahr, A. and Payne, L. J. (1992). *Immunobiology* **184**, 126–146.

Manthorpe, M., Cornefert-Jensen, F., Hartikka, J., Felgner J., Rundell, A., Margalith, M. and Dwarki, V. (1993). *Hum. Gene Ther.* **4**, 419–431.

McCoy, J. and LaVallie, E. R. (1994). In *Current Protocols in Molecular Biology* (F. M. Ausubel *et al.*, eds), Unit 16.8, pp. 16.8.1–16.8.14. Current Protocols Publishing, New York.

Mizukani, T., Komatsu, Y., Hosoi, N., Itoh, S. and Tetsuo, O. (1986). *Biotech. Lett.* **8**, 605–610.

Montgomery, D. L., Donnelly, J. J., Shiver, J. W., Liu, M. A. and Ulmer, J. B. (1994). *Curr. Opin. Biotechnol.* **5**, 505–510.

Murphy, C. I. and Pirvnica-Worms, H. (1994). In *Current Protocols in Molecular Biology* (F. M. Ausubel *et al.*, eds), Unit 16.9, pp. 16.9.1–16.9.6. Current Protocols Publishing, New York.

Nabel, G. J., Nabel, E. G., Yang, Z. Y., Fox, B. A., Plautz, G. E., Gao, X., Huang, L., Shu, S., Gordon, D. and Chang, A. E. (1993). *Proc. Natl. Acad. Sci. USA* **90**, 11307–11311.

O'Reilly, D. R., Miller, L. K. and Kuchow, V. A. (1992). In *Baculovirus Expression Vectors: A Laboratory Manual*, pp. 1–347. W.H. Freeman, New York.

Pati, U.K. (1992). *Gene* **114**, 285–288.

Schein, D. H. (1989). *Bio/Technology* **7**, 1141–1148.

Smith, D. B. (1993). *Methods Mol. Cell Biol.* **4**, 220–229.

Smith, D. B. and Corcoran, L. M. (1994). In *Current Protocols in Molecular Biology* (F.M. Ausubel *et al.*, eds), Unit 16.7, pp. 16.7.1–16.7.7. Current Protocols Publishing, New York.

Smith, D. B., Davern, K. M., Board, P. G., Tiu, W. U., Garcia, E. G. and Mitchell, G. F. (1986). *Proc. Natl. Acad. Sci. USA* **83**, 8703–8707.

Stuber, D., Matile, H. and Garotta, G. (1990). *Immunol. Methods* **4**, 121–152.

Tang, D. C., Devit, M. and Johnston, S. A. (1992). *Nature* **356**, 152–154.

Taussig, R., Quarmby, L. and Gilman, A. (1993). *J. Biol. Chem.* **268**, 9–12.

Ulmer, J. B., Donnelly, J. J., Parker, S. E., Rhodes, G. H., Felgner, P. L., Dwarki, V. J., Gromkowski, S. H., Deck, R. R., Dewitt, C. M., Friedman, A. *et. al.* (1993). *Science* **259**, 1745–1749.

Wang, B., Ugen, K. E., Srikantan, V., Agadjanyan, M. G., Dang, K., Refaeli, Y., Sato, A. I., Williams, W. V. and Weiner, D. B. (1993). *Proc. Natl. Acad. Sci. USA* **90**, 4156–4160.

Wolff, J. A., Ludtke, J. J., Acsadi, G., Williams, P. and Jani, A. (1992). *Hum. Mol. Genet.* **1**, 363–369.

7

The GABA$_A$ Receptor Gene Family as Targets for Drug Discovery

P. J. WHITING, K. L. HADINGHAM, P. B. WINGROVE, E. GARRETT, K. QUIRK, K. A. WAFFORD, C. I. RAGAN and R. M. MCKERNAN

Neuroscience Research Centre, Merck Sharp and Dohme Research Laboratories, Harlow, Essex, CM20 2QR, UK

Abstract

The GABA$_A$ receptor is an excellent example of a drug target which has entered a new phase of attention from pharmaceutical companies as a result of discoveries brought about by molecular genetic approaches. GABA (γ-aminobutyric acid) is a neurotransmitter which inhibits neuronal activity throughout the central nervous system by activating the GABA$_A$ receptor, a multisubunit transmembrane protein, opening an integral chloride channel which results in a hyperpolarization of the nerve cell membrane. The GABA$_A$ receptor is the site of action of a number of clinically important drugs which have been available for many years as anxiolytics (e.g. benzodiazepines such as valium), hypnotics (sleeping pills) and anticonvulsants. These drugs act allosterically at modulatory sites on the GABA$_A$ receptor to increase its activity. They are however far from perfect, having a number of side effects including sedation, tolerance, dependence and interaction with alcohol. Thus there is clearly room for improvement.

Until 1987 it was thought that GABA$_A$ receptors consisted of two subtypes, so-called BZ1 and BZ2, defined by their affinities for certain benzodiazepine ligands. Work primarily from the laboratories of Barnard and Seeburg (see Macdonald and Olsen, 1994, for review), as well as others, turned this idea upside down. Using protein purification and microsequencing followed by cDNA cloning, the cDNA sequences of two GABA$_A$ receptor polypeptides were identified. This was only the beginning: low stringency hybridization cDNA library screening approaches allowed the isolation of a family of GABA$_A$ receptor subunit cDNAs which in the

GENOMES, MOLECULAR BIOLOGY AND DRUG DISCOVERY
ISBN 0-12-137790-3

mammalian brain currently total 13. These have been divided into subgroups according to their relative sequence homology: $\alpha1-\alpha6$, $\beta1-\beta3$, $\gamma1-\gamma3$, δ. Numerous questions arise from this discovery which are fundamental to any drug discovery programme wishing to exploit these new findings. How are these subunits arranged *in vivo* to form receptor subtypes? In which regions of the brain are they expressed? Can we accurately genetically reconstitute the receptors in recombinant systems? What are the functional and pharmacological properties of the receptor subtypes? What are the physiological roles of each receptor subtype, and which are good targets for a new generation of drugs acting at $GABA_A$ receptor subtypes? We have utilized a molecular approach to begin to answer some of these questions, and these data will be presented.

1 Introduction to the GABA$_A$ receptor

Gamma-aminobutyric acid (GABA) is the major inhibitory neurotransmitter in the vertebrate central nervous system (CNS). It is localized at many synapses throughout the CNS where it modulates the inhibitory tone by activating two classes of neurotransmitter receptor, $GABA_A$ and $GABA_B$. The latter are thought to be G-protein linked receptors, acting by activation of second messenger systems within the cell. $GABA_A$ receptors are ligand gated ion channels which mediate fast inhibitory neurotransmission (Macdonald and Olsen, 1994). The binding of the agonist, GABA, to the $GABA_A$ receptor results in allosteric changes in the receptor structure over a rapid (millisecond) time scale, leading to transient (millisecond) opening of an intrinsic ion channel. The ion channel is permeable to anions (primarily chloride) which flow down their concentration gradient into the cell, leading to a hyperpolarization of the cell membrane, dampening any excitatory (depolarizing) events at that particular synapse.

The $GABA_A$ receptor is a pharmacologically very rich macromolecule. In addition to the agonist (GABA) binding site, several additional ligand binding sites have been identified, through which a range of pharmacologically active agents have been shown to modulate the function of the receptor by allosterically promoting or inhibiting the action of GABA. These modulatory agents include ethanol and neurosteroids, as well as some clinically important drugs, most notably the benzodiazepines (BZ) and barbiturates (for review see Doble and Martin, 1992; Macdonald and Olsen; 1994; Whiting *et al.*, 1995). General anaesthetics such as halothane may also exert their activity through the $GABA_A$ receptor. All these drugs bind to unique allosteric sites on the $GABA_A$ receptor and potentiate the action of GABA. At the molecular level, BZs are known to increase the frequency of opening of the chloride channel, while barbiturates act by increasing the time for which the chloride channel stays open. The net effect is an increased hyperpolarization of the nerve cell membrane and dampening of nerve cell firing. BZs, or more correctly, compounds which act at the BZ binding site, are some of the most widely utilized drugs. They are prescribed as anxiolytics (treatment of anxiety), hypnotics (sedatives) and anticonvulsants. Perhaps the most widely known BZ is the Hoffman-La Roche drug Valium (diazepam). It is a testament to the safety of these drugs that they have been so widely used as therapeutic agents since they were first introduced in 1960. However they are not perfect drugs, suffering from a number of side effects including sedation (a requirement for a hypnotic, but not for treatment of anxiety), interaction with alcohol, and a tendency to tolerance and dependence with long-term use. It is thus clear that there is room for improvement in terms of their side effect profile.

2 The GABA_A receptor gene family

Until 1987 the nature of the GABA_A receptor/BZ binding site complex had been defined using pharmacological and biochemical techniques. The receptor could be characterized pharmacologically by radioligand binding using radiolabelled BZ site ligands. Through this approach it became clear that GABA_A receptors in membranes prepared from mammalian brain were not a homogeneous population, but could be divided into two populations, so-called BZ1 and BZ2, the former having higher affinity for certain BZ site ligands, such as the Lederle compound Cl218,872 (Squires et al., 1979). This was the first indication that there may be subtypes of GABA_A receptors.

It was not until the tools of modern molecular biology were exploited that the extent of heterogeneity within the GABA_A receptor became clear. Enough receptor protein was purified from bovine brain to allow amino acid microsequencing of receptor polypeptides. Oligonucleotide probes were designed from these amino acid sequences which were used to screen a brain cDNA library. cDNAs encoding two polypeptides of 456 and 474 amino acids were initially identified, referred to as α1 and β1 (Schofield et al., 1987). This was a breakthrough in our understanding of the GABA_A receptor. In terms of members of the GABA_A receptor family it turned out to be only the tip of the iceberg. Using low stringency hybridization techniques, probes based upon the α1 and β1 subunit cDNAs were used to screen brain cDNA libraries. A family of GABA_A receptor polypeptide cDNAs was subsequently identified. These have been subdivided according to their relative amino acid sequence identities into α (α1–α6), β (β1–β3), γ (γ1–γ3) and δ subunits (for review see Whiting et al., 1995). Within each subgroup there is 70–80% sequence identity, whereas between subgroups there is 30–40%. Initially, bovine and rodent cDNAs were isolated and characterized. We, and others, have now cloned and sequenced cDNAs encoding human GABA_A receptor subunits (Schofield et al., 1989; Pritchett et al., 1989a,b; Ymer et al., 1989; Wagstaff et al., 1991; Wingrove et al., 1991; Hadingham et al., 1993a,b; Whiting, unpublished). The homology of the human deduced amino acid sequences with the rodent equivalents varies from only one amino acid difference (the α1 subunit; Schofield et al., 1989) to 62 differences (the α4 subunit; Whiting, unpublished). The deduced amino acid sequences of the GABA_A receptor subunits exhibit sequence identity (20–30%) with the nicotinic acetylcholine receptor, the glycine receptor and the 5-hydroxytryptamine-3 (5-HT_3) receptor. The GABA_A receptor is thus a member of an extended ligand gated ion channel superfamily, and by analogy it would be predicted to be a pentameric structure, with subunits arranged around a central ion channel (Unwin, 1989).

The discovery of a family of GABA_A receptors allows the possibility of targeting BZ-type modulatory drugs to one particular receptor subtype, avoiding perhaps the side effects of these compounds described above. It also raises a whole range of questions which are fundamental to any drug discovery programme wishing to exploit these new findings. How are these subunits arranged *in vivo* to form receptor subtypes, and where in the CNS are they expressed? Can we accurately genetically reconstitute these receptor subtypes in recombinant systems? What are the pharmacological properties of these receptor subtypes? What are the physiological roles for each receptor subtype, and which are the targets for a new generation of drugs?

3 The composition of GABA_A receptors *in vivo*

By either expressing recombinant receptor subunit combinations in *Xenopus* oocytes or transiently transfected mammalian cells it soon became clear that to reconstitute a receptor with the pharmacological and functional properties of a native receptor required an α, a β and a γ subunit (Pritchett *et al.*, 1989a). However, this still meant that if each receptor were to contain at least one of each α, β and γ the theoretical number of subtypes would be 9126 ($6 \times 3 \times 3 \times 13 \times 13$). From our knowledge of the related nicotinic acetylcholine receptor it is likely that the subunit assembly is structurally constrained, and thus the actual number of receptor subtypes is only a fraction of the theoretical number.

To investigate the subunit structure of native GABA_A receptor subtypes we have generated a panel of subunit-specific antibodies. The domain of each subunit between putative transmembrane spanning regions TM3 and TM4 is the most divergent and thus contains sequences suitable for generation of subunit specific-antibodies. To achieve this, cDNA sequences encoding amino acid sequences (50–80 residues in length) from this region of each subunit were genetically engineered into the bacterial expression vector pRSET5a. Milligram amounts of recombinant proteins were generated and used to immunize rabbits: the antisera were subunit specific, high titre and high affinity (McKernan *et al.*, 1991). The advantages of using longer recombinant polypeptides as opposed to short (10–15 residues in length) synthetic peptides are that there are more epitopes available which should result in a higher titre antisera, and that the longer the sequence the more likely that epitopes will be exposed on the surface on the receptor macromolecule in its native state and thus accessible in immunoprecipitation studies.

To investigate the combinations of subunits which exist in native GABA_A receptors, two types of experiments were carried out. In the first, receptors solubilized from rat brain membranes with detergent were quantitatively immunoprecipitated with subunit-specific antisera, either alone or in pairs. The immunoprecipitated receptors were radiolabelled with [^{3}H]muscimol (which binds to the GABA recognition site and is considered to label all GABA_A receptors) or a BZ site radioligand. The rationale is that two subunits exist in the same receptor molecule if the sum of the proportion of receptors immunoprecipitated by two antisera together is significantly less than the total of the proportion of receptors immunoprecipitated individually by each antiserum. The second approach utilizes immunopurification of detergent-solubilized receptors followed by Western blot analysis, i.e. purification of receptors using antibody to subunit x, followed by Western blot analysis using antibodies to subunit y. While this second method is not quantitative it does quite definitively demonstrate the presence of two subunit types within a receptor macromolecule.

The data obtained from studies described above (McKernan *et al.*, 1991; Quirk *et al.*, 1994a,b), together with information derived from other laboratories which have used subunit-specific antibodies (Duggan and Stephenson, 1990; Benke *et al.*, 1991; Duggan *et al.*, 1992; for review see Whiting *et al.*, 1995) or *in situ* hybridization techniques (Wisden *et al.*, 1992) to look at the expression patterns of receptor subunits, have been collated into a model of the *major* GABA_A receptor subtypes which exist in the rat brain (Fig. 1). The least well defined are the β subunits, probably because they have a very high degree of sequence identity and it has thus proven more difficult to develop useful specific antisera against the β subunit. Our current model suggests that the number of major subtypes is relatively small. This does of course not discount the existence of a number of minor receptor populations. The most abundant receptor population is $\alpha1\beta2\gamma2$. Analysis of the BZ pharmacology of these immunoprecipitated receptors indicates that they represent the BZ1 subtype (McKernan *et al.*, 1991). The next most abundant populations are $\alpha2\beta\gamma2$ and $\alpha3\beta\gamma2$. Analysis of the BZ pharmacology of these receptors indicates that they represent the BZ2 subtype (McKernan *et al.*, 1991). The $\alpha5$ subunit is found primarily in the hippocampus, where there is evidence that it is found as an $\alpha5\beta\gamma2$ or perhaps $\alpha5\beta\gamma2\gamma3$ complex. The $\alpha6$ subunit is expressed only in the cerebellum, where it is found as

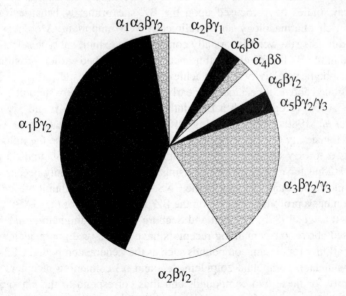

Fig. 1 Model of GABA_A receptor composition in whole rat brain.

α6βγ2 and α6βδ (Quirk *et al.*, 1994a). The former of these has a high affinity BZ binding site, while the latter does not. The γ1 subunit appears to be primarily assembled with the α2 subunit (Quirk *et al.*, 1994b), though as a minor population. There is some evidence that receptors can contain more than one type of a subunit (McKernan *et al.*, 1991; Pollard *et al.*, 1993), although in some cases this is in dispute (Quirk *et al.*, 1994a). There is also some evidence that some receptors can contain more than one type of γ subunit (Quirk *et al.*, 1994b).

Data from *in situ* hybridization and immunolocalization studies have demonstrated very distinct patterns of expression of the receptor subunits throughout the CNS (Wisden *et al.*, 1992; Laurie *et al.*, 1992; Fritschy *et al.*, 1992). It is becoming clear that the expression of these receptor subunits, and thus receptor subtypes, is tightly controlled in both a spatial and temporal manner.

4 Expression and characterization of recombinant human GABA$_A$ receptors

We have utilized three different systems to express recombinant human GABA$_A$ receptors: *Xenopus* oocytes, transiently transfected mammalian cells, and stably transfected mammalian cells. *Xenopus* oocytes are a useful system for measuring by electrophysiology the function of recombinant receptors, and the effects of drugs (e.g. the efficacy of modulatory compounds such as BZs). Transiently transfected cells are useful for preliminary pharmacological characterization of receptor subtypes and for structure–function analyses using site-directed mutagenesis. Stably transfected cells are our system of choice for both detailed pharmacological analysis and production of recombinant receptor for drug screening programmes. Most pharmacological studies have focused upon the BZ site primarily because it has an extremely rich pharmacology and is clinically very important. Moreover, drugs which bind to this site were historically considered to exhibit subtype selectivity as manifested in the BZ1–BZ2 classical nomenclature described earlier, providing evidence that subtype selectivity may be achievable through this site.

As mentioned above, it became clear early on that the minimum subunit composition of a GABA$_A$ receptor with a BZ binding site was an α, a β and a γ subunit (Pritchett *et al.*, 1989a). By expressing different subunit combinations in *Xenopus* oocytes or transiently transfected cells it was possible to determine the influence of the various α, β or γ subunits on the affinities of a range of compounds at the BZ site. Most studies have been performed using the γ2 subunit, mainly because this is by far the most abundant γ subunit in the CNS. The type of α subunit present in the combination has a profound effect upon the BZ pharmacology of the GABA$_A$ receptor (Pritchett *et al.*, 1989b; Pritchett and Seeburg, 1990; Hadingham *et al.*, 1993a). As discussed above, α1-containing receptors have a BZ1-type pharmacology, having higher affinity for certain compounds such as the Lederle compound CL218, 872 and the Synthelabo compound zolpidem. α2- and α3-containing receptors have a lower affinity for these two compounds and thus correspond to the classical BZ2 binding site. α5-containing receptors have an even lower affinity for zolpidem, and thus do not fit into the BZ1–BZ2 pharmacological nomenclature. α1-, α2-, α3- and α5- containing receptors all have high affinity for classical BZs such as diazepam. α4- and α6- containing receptors are unique in having a very low affinity for diazepam (Luddens *et al.*, 1990; Wisden *et al.*, 1991). This complexity is somewhat simplified when the influence of the β subunit on the BZ pharmacology of GABA$_A$ receptor subtypes is examined. The type of β subunit present (β1, β2 or β3) in a GABA$_A$ receptor has no detectable influence upon the BZ pharmacology (Hadingham *et al.*, 1993b). Finally, the type of γ subunit present (γ1, γ2 or γ3), like the α subunit, has a major influence upon the BZ pharmacology of the GABA$_A$ receptor (Ymer *et al.*, 1990; Wafford *et al.*, 1993; Luddens *et al.*, 1994). From this data it is obvious the classical BZ1–BZ2 nomenclature is no longer appropriate, and that GABA$_A$ receptors must be classified according to their molecular composition.

There are other modulatory sites on the GABA$_A$ receptor in addition to the BZ site. Pharmacological characterization of these sites on different receptor subunit combinations has been less rigorous. However, for the barbiturate site and the neurosteriod modulatory sites there is not a great deal of evidence for subtype selectivity (Puia *et al.*, 1990; Shingai *et al.*, 1991; Hadingham *et al.*, 1993b). Thus, when considering the classical modulatory sites on the GABA$_A$ receptor it is clear that the BZ site holds the most promise for the development of novel subtype selective drugs.

To enable the development of drugs which are selective for a particular receptor subtype it is necessary to be able to express recombinant receptors *in vitro* in relatively large amounts, and in a form that is essentially indistinguishable from that of the native receptor. The choice of which subunits to co-express to form receptor subtypes is determined by the detailed biochemical and pharmacological analyses described above. For this purpose we have developed a series of transfected mammalian cell lines stably expressing recombinant human GABA$_A$ receptor subtypes (Hadingham *et al.*, 1992, 1993b). The eukaryotic expression vector we have utilized (pMSGneo) has the mouse mammary tumour virus promoter for control of expression of the receptor subunits. This promoter is steroid inducible, such that transcription of the cDNA, and therefore receptor expression, occurs only when dexamethasone is added to the culture medium of the transfected cells. This inducible system was chosen because of the concern that constitutive expression of an exogenous chloride channel in the transfected cells (mouse fibroblast L cells) would be toxic. Stable integration of three subunit cDNAs is achieved by co-transfection of three expression vector constructs each containing α subunit cDNA (an α, a β and a γ subunit), and analysing transfected cells for high affinity binding of a radioligand for the BZ site since we know that reconstitution of a fully functional receptor requires correct assembly of an α, a β and a γ subunit. These stably transfected cell lines express in the range of 1 pmol of [^{3}H]BZ binding sites (i.e. about a picomole of receptors assuming one BZ binding site per receptor molecule) per mg protein. Detailed biochemical, pharmacological and functional analyses have demonstrated that when an α, a β and a γ subunit are co-expressed in these stably transfected cells they preferentially co-assemble together to form receptors which have all of the properties expected of native $GABA_A$ receptors (Hadingham *et al.*, 1992; Horne *et al.*, 1992, 1993). This is, of course, an absolute requirement.

5 Identification of novel drug binding sites

The characterization of drug targets at the molecular level not only leads to greater insights of existing drug binding sites, but can reveal the existence of hitherto unrecognized pharmacological sites. An example of this is the loreclezole binding site on the $GABA_A$ receptor. Until recently the molecular basis for the anticonvulsant action of loreclezole, a compound synthesized by Jannsens, was unknown but thought to be via a GABAergic mechanism. By examining its effect on recombinant human $GABA_A$ receptors expressed in *Xenopus* oocytes we were able to demonstrate that loreclezole acted by allosterically potentiating the action of GABA (Wafford *et al.*, 1994). It does not act at the same site as BZs, however, but through a novel modulatory site located on the β subunit. Indeed, loreclezole is a subtype selective compound, having approximately 300-fold higher affinity for $GABA_A$ receptors containing a β2 or β3 subunit over receptors containing a β1 subunit (Wafford *et al.*, 1994). The loreclezole modulatory site is thus a novel pharmacological target which could be exploited to develop $GABA_A$ receptor subtype-selective drugs.

6 Determination of the function of $GABA_A$ receptor subtypes

The discovery of the existence of a family of $GABA_A$ receptor subtypes expressed throughout the CNS leads to the obvious question: what is their function? This question has more than one perspective. Firstly, an understanding of the physiological roles of each subtype in neurotransmission will inevitably contribute to a greater understanding of the function of the brain. Secondly, if we are to identify a particular receptor subtype as a target for a selective drug, understanding of what that subtype does would be invaluable information. This reasoning applies whether we are aiming to develop a novel drug which lacks the undesirable side effects of existing non-selective drugs, or whether we are aiming to develop a drug for a new indication. There are several ways one could go about answering this question, including: (i) use antisense approaches (e.g. oligonucleotides or viral delivery to the brain of antisense DNA constructs) specifically to down-regulate expression of a receptor subunit and analyse the effects in animal models; (ii) use transgenic approaches to overexpress or knock out selected subunits, and characterize the phenotype in animal models; (iii) characterize the phenotypes of naturally occurring mutations, such as strains of mice lacking a receptor subunit (Culiat *et al.*, 1994); and (iv) develop subtype-selective compounds (agonists or antagonists) and characterize their effects in animal models.

7 Conclusions

Our understanding of the GABA$_A$ receptor has changed greatly over the last few years. Revelation of the existence of a GABA$_A$ receptor gene family did not come from human genome sequencing programmes but from the application of molecular biological approaches. Nevertheless, the approaches and issues discussed in this chapter will certainly apply to many of the new proteins identified by genome sequencing, whether they be additional members of known gene families, or completely novel entities. In the future it is likely that the 'rate-limiting step' will not be identification of cDNA sequences, but characterization and determination of the function of the proteins themselves.

References

Benke, D., Mertens, S., Trzeciak, A., Gillesen, D. and Mohler, H. (1991). *J Biol. Chem.* **266**, 4478–4483.

Culiat, C. T., Stubbs, L. J., Montgomery, C. S., Russell, L. B. and Rinchik, E. M. (1994). *Proc. Natl. Acad. Sci. USA* **91**, 2815–2819.

Doble, A. and Martin, I. L. (1992). *Trends. Pharmacol. Sci.* **1992**, 76–81.

Duggan, M. J. and Stephenson, F. A. (1990). *J. Biol. Chem.* **265**, 3831–3835.

Duggan, M., Pollard, S. and Stephenson, F. A. (1992). *J. Neurochem.* **58**, 72–77.

Fritschy, J. M., Benke, D., Mertens, S., Gao, B. and Mohler H. (1992). *Proc. Natl. Acad. Sci. USA* **89**, 6726–6730.

Hadingham, K. L., Harkness, P. C., McKernan, R. M., Quirk, K., Le Bourdelles, B., Horne, A. L., Kemp, J. A., Barnard, E. A.,Ragan C. I. and Whiting, P. J. (1992). *Proc. Natl. Acad. Sci. USA* **89**, 6378–6382.

Hadingham, K. L., Wingrove, P., Le Bourdelles, B., Palmer, K. J., Ragan, C. I. and Whiting, P. J. (1993a). *Mol. Pharmacol.* **43**, 970–975.

Hadingham, K. L., Wingrove, P. B., Wafford, K. A. C. Bain, Kemp, J. A., Palmer, K. J., Wilson, A. W., Wilcox, A. S., Sikela, J. M., Ragan, C.I. and Whiting, P. J. (1993b). *Mol. Pharmacol.* **44**, 1211–1218.

Horne, A. L., Hadingham, K. L., Macauley, A. J., Whiting, P. J. and Kemp, J. A. (1992). *Br. J. Pharmacol.* **107**, 732–737.

Horne A. L., Harkness P. C., Hadingham K. L., Whiting P. and Kemp J. A. (1993). *Br. J. Pharmacol.* **108**, 711–716.

Laurie, D. J., Seeburg, P. H. and Wisden, W. (1992). *J. Neurosci.* **12**, 1063–1076.

Luddens, H., Pritchett, D. B., Kohler, M., Killisch, I., Keinanen, K., Monyer, H., Sprengel, R. and Seeburg, P. H. (1990). *Nature* **346**, 648–651.

Luddens, H., Seeburg, P. H. and Korpi, E. R. (1994). *Mol. Pharmacol.* **45**, 810–814.

Macdonald, R. L. and Olsen, R. W. (1994). *Annu. Rev. Neurosci.* **17**, 569–602.

McKernan, R. M., Quirk, K., Prince, R., Cox, P. A.,Gillard, N. P., Ragan, C. I. and Whiting, P. J. (1991). *Neuron* **7**, 667–676.

Pollard, S., Duggan, M.J. and Stephenson, F.A. (1993). *J. Biol Chem.* **268**, 3753–3757.

Pritchett, D. B. and Seeburg, P. H. (1990). *J. Neurochem.* **54**, 1802–1804.

Pritchett, D. B., Sontheimer, H., Shivers, B. H., Ymer, S., Kettenmann, H., Schofield, P. H. and Seeburg, P. H. (1989a). *Nature* **338**, 582–585.

Pritchett D.B., Luddens H. and Seeburg P.H. (1989b). *Science* **245**, 1389–1392.

Puia, G., Santi, M., Vicini, S., Pritchett, D. B., Purdy, R. H., Paul, S. M., Seeburg, P. H. and Costa, E. (1990). *Neuron* **4**, 759–765.

Quirk, K., Gillard N. P., Ragan C. I., Whiting P. J. and McKernan R. M. (1994a). *J. Biol. Chem.* **269**, 16020-16028.

Quirk, K., Gillard, N. P., Ragan, C. I., Whiting, P. J. and McKernan, R. M. (1994b). *Mol. Pharmacol.* **45**, 1061–1070.

Schofield, P. R., Darlison, M. G., Fujita, N., Burt, D. R., Stephenson, F. A., Rodriguez, H., Rhee, L. M., Ramachandran, J., Reale, V., Glencourse, T. A., Seeburg, P. H. and Barnard, E. A. (1987). *Nature* **328**, 221–227.

Schofield, P. R., Pritchett, D. B., Sontheimer, H., Kettenmann, H. and Seeburg, P. H. (1989). *FEBS Lett.* **244**, 361–364.

Shingai, R., Sutherland, M. L. and Barnard, E. A. (1991). *Eur. J. Pharmacol.* **206**, 77–80.

Squires, R. F., Benson, D. I., Braestrup, C., Coupet, J., Myers, V. and Beer, B. (1979). *Pharmacol. Biochem. Behav.* **10**, 825–830.

Unwin, N. (1989). *Neuron* **3**, 565–575.

Wafford, K. A., Bain, C. J., Whiting, P. J. and Kemp, J. A. (1993). *Mol. Pharmacol.* **44**, 437–442.

Wafford, K. A., Bain, C. J., Quirk, K., McKernan, R. M., Wingrove, P. B., Whiting, P. J. and Kemp, J. A. (1994). *Neuron* **12**, 775–782.

Wagstaff, J., Chaillet, J. R. and Lalande, M. (1991). *Genomics* **11**, 1071–1078.

Whiting, P. J., McKernan, R. M. and Wafford, K. A. (1995). *Int. Rev. Neurobiol.* (in press).

Wingrove, P., Hadingham, K., Wafford, K., Kemp, J. A., Ragan, C. I. and Whiting, P. (1991). *Biochem. Soc. Trans.* **20**, 17S.

Wisden, W., Herb, A., Weiland, H., Keinanen, K., Luddens, H. and Seeburg, P. H. (1991). *FEBS Lett.* **289**, 227–230.

Wisden, W., Laurie, D. J., Monyer, H. M. and Seeburg, P. H. (1992). *J. Neurosci.* **12**, 1040–1062.

Ymer, S., Schofield, P. R., Draguhn, A., Werner, P., Kohler, M. and Seeburg, P. H. (1989). *EMBO J.* **8**, 1665–1670.

Ymer, S., Draguhn, A., Wisden, W., Werner, P., Keinanen, K., Schofield, P. R., Sprengel, R., Pritchett, D. B. and Seeburg, P. H. (1990). *EMBO J.* **9**, 3261–3267.

8

Drug Discovery and the Transcriptional Control of the Human Beta Globin Gene Locus

F. GROSVELD[1,2], M. ANTONIOU[1], M. BERRY[1],
E. de BOER[2], N. DILLON[1], D. DRABEK[2],
J. ELLIS[1], P. FRASER[2], J. HALEY[3],
S. PHILIPSEN[2], S. PRUZINA[2],
S. RAGUZ–BOLOGNESI[1], D. SMITH[3],
T. TRIMBORN[2] and M. WIJGERDE[2]

[1] MRC National Institute for Medical Research, The Ridgeway, Mill Hill, London NW7 1AA, UK
[2] MGC Department of Cell Biology and Genetics, Erasmus University Rotterdam, PO Box 1738, 3000 DR, Rotterdam, The Netherlands
[3] Oncogene Science, 106 Charles Lindbergh Boulevard, Uniondale, NY 11553, USA

Abstract

Sickle cell anaemia and thalassaemia are among the most widespread fatal genetic diseases. They are found in people from all areas of the world that have been infested with malaria, including southern Europe. Worldwide 240 million people are heterozygous for these haemoglobinopathies. Each year 20 000–40 000 children are born with β-thalassaemias and 100 000 children, particularly in the black population, are born with homozygous sickle cell anaemia. β-Thalassaemia and sickle cell anaemia are caused by genetic lesions which result in the absence, decrease or mutation of β-globin chains. β-Globin chains together with the α-globin chains and haem form haemoglobin, the main constituent of red blood cells, responsible for delivering oxygen to all the tissues. The treatment of these diseases is at present inadequate, very expensive and unsatisfactory for several reasons. There is an urgent need for novel treatments, and our aim is the construction of mouse models which can be used to develop a non-gene therapy approach. The β-like globin genes are present as a multigene cluster on the short arm of human chromosome 11. The cluster contains

GENOMES, MOLECULAR BIOLOGY AND DRUG DISCOVERY
ISBN 0-12-137790-3

five genes arranged in the same order as they are expressed during development. It is known that expression of a fetal haemoglobin gene in the affected cells of patients with β-thalassaemia or sickle cell anaemia mutations will prevent the development of the disease. We are constructing transgenic mice and cell lines which will carry a modified human β-globin gene domain. These will be used to screen robotically for novel therapeutic compounds that will increase the amount of fetal haemoglobin expression. In addition, we are constructing transgenic mice which model human sickle cell anaemia. These mice will be used to study the pathophysiology of the disease and to test the aforementioned compounds for their ability to increase fetal haemoglobin expression and ameliorate sickle cell disease.

1 Introduction

α-Globin and β-globin polypeptides are subunits of the tetrameric oxygen binding protein haemoglobin which transports oxygen throughout the body. The β-like globin genes are present as a multigene cluster on the short arm of human chromosome 11. The cluster contains five active genes arranged in the same order as they are expressed during development (Fig. 1). The embryonic ε-globin gene is located at the 5' end and is expressed in yolk sac-derived erythroid cells during the first weeks of gestation. The γ-globin genes are expressed in yolk sac and fetal liver-derived erythrocytes up to birth. At the 3' end are the adult δ- and β-globin genes which are first activated in the fetal liver and increased in expression after birth, when the site of haematopoiesis shifts to the adult bone marrow. The expression of the δ-globin gene is low, only a few per cent of that of the β-globin gene. Hence mutations in both alleles of the β-globin gene will lead to abnormalities such as thalassaemia or sickle cell anaemia only after birth.

β-Thalassaemia is caused by the absence (or decrease) of β-globin chains which causes an imbalance in the α- to β-globin chain ratio resulting in precipitation of untetramerized α-chains and consequent cell damage. More than a hundred different mutations which affect β-globin expression have been identified. Most of these are point mutations which affect the transcription, splicing or translation of β-globin mRNA, resulting in a lack or decrease in β-globin synthesis and early destruction of the red cells. Sickle cell anaemia is the result of one amino acid change in the β-globin protein (βs). This aggregates under low oxygen conditions and causes the cells to adopt a characteristic sickle shape. The sickled cells cause blockages in microcapillaries leading to crises and tissue necrosis. The treatment of these diseases involves either pain control alone (for βs) or pain control supplemented by regular administration of blood transfusion in combination with iron chelation therapy, which is unsatisfactory for several reasons. It is inadequate, very expensive (tens of thousands of dollars per year per patient) and involves large amounts of blood with all its associated risks of infection. An alternative and curative treatment is bone marrow transplantation, but this requires transplantation between individuals with all the problems associated with donor/recipient matching. Interestingly, in certain individuals additional mutations can lead to elevated expression of the fetal γ-globin genes

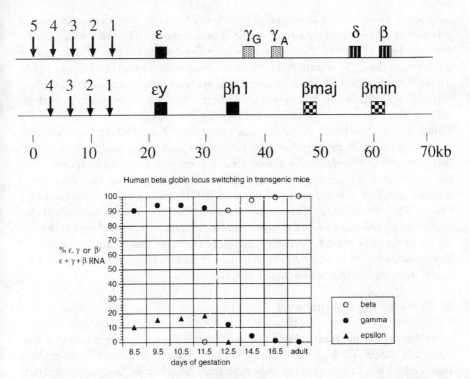

Fig. 1 The human and mouse β-globin locus. The top line shows the human β-globin locus. The five arrows indicate the position of the LCR containing the hypersensitive regions HS1–5. These regions bind a number of erythroid-specific and ubiquitous transcription factors. The second line shows the mouse ß-globin locus. Distances are given in kilobases (kb). The panel at the bottom shows the expression of the human genes when the human entire β-globin locus is introduced into transgenic mice (Strouboulis *et al.*, 1992).

after birth (hereditary persistence of fetal haemoglobin, HPFH) and as a result, the effects of the mutation in the β-globin gene are greatly ameliorated (for review, see Wood *et al.*, 1993). The HPFH mutations can be divided into two groups, namely promoter mutations that appear to suppress silencing (Berry *et al.*, 1992) and deletions in the locus which appear to override silencing by placing an enhancer sequence close to the γ-globin genes (Anagnou *et al.*, 1995). In terms of drug development, the promoter mutations are at present the most interesting, because they may provide a direct way into the discovery of novel compounds that may interfere directly with the regulation of the silencing process.

It is therefore important to understand which regulatory regions are involved in globin gene expression and what assays could be used to study or assay the regulatory process. To the 5′ side of the ε gene is the so-called locus control region (LCR, Fig. 1), which contains a large number of transcription factor binding sites and is required for the expression of all the β-like genes *in vivo*. Linkage of this region to either α- or β-globin genes followed by introduction of these genes into transgenic mice leads to expression at normal physiological levels, independent of the site of integration of the DNA construct in the mouse genome (Grosveld *et al.*, 1987; Hanscombe *et al.*, 1989). This property is maintained when the entire β-globin gene cluster with the LCR is introduced into transgenic mice (Strouboulis *et al.*, 1992). The results show that the genes are expressed at endogenous gene levels, are appropriately regulated during development, and completely free from unwanted position effects. The ε gene is expressed in the embryo and suppressed at the time of the switch to the fetal liver, mimicking the expression of the endogenous mouse εy gene. Expression of the γ-globin gene mimics the embryonic specific endogenous βh1 gene, but in contrast to the mouse gene, it is only suppressed around day 16 in the fetal liver of transgenic mice (Fig. 1; for review see Dillon and Grosveld, 1993) unless a mutation is introduced which causes HPFH, both in humans and mice (see below; Berry *et al.*, 1992). The mouse therefore represents an excellent model system to study and manipulate the expression of introduced human globin genes and we are using this system for different approaches to novel treatments for the haemoglobinopathies. The two that will be discussed in particular are gene therapy and the use of transcription modulation to aid drug discovery.

2 Vectors for gene therapy

Gene therapy for the haemoglobinopathies requires the stable integration of a normal, fully functional β-globin transcription unit into the genome of bone marrow stem cells. This, at present, can only efficiently be achieved using retroviral and adeno-associated virus (AAV) vectors. The feasibility of such an approach employing retroviral vectors was first demonstrated in mouse model systems as long ago as the late 1980s (Dzierzak *et al.*, 1988). However, a number of major obstacles remain in the way of the general use of these viral vectors for gene therapy applications. Firstly, the amount of DNA that can be accommodated within these vectors is small; approximately 8 kb for retroviruses and 4.4 kb for AAV. Therefore, the therapeutic transcription unit must be reduced in size without significantly impeding its function, so that it can be accommodated within the virus. Another problem is that the replacement of the viral genetic material with the gene of choice almost invariably results in a marked reduction in the efficiency of virus production. Thus, the therapeutic transcription unit has to be constructed in such a fashion as to have a minimal detrimental effect on viral titre. This again is something that can only be addressed empirically, requiring the testing of many candidate constructs before an optimized transcription unit is obtained (Sadelain *et al.*, 1995).

Another important consideration is that once integration into bone marrow stem cells is achieved, the β-globin transcription unit must function at a sufficiently high and sustained level in differentiated red cells to be of therapeutic value. It is known from patients with β-thalassaemia intermedia, that a level of β-globin which is 25% of normal is adequate to provide transfusion independence. The level of β- or γ-globin that is required to prevent sickling in sickle cell disease is not known exactly, but is likely to be comparable to that for thalassaemia. It therefore follows that a single copy, β-globin transgene delivered via a retroviral or AAV vector into a given stem cell must function at a minimum of 50% of the wild type level of expression to produce a therapeutic amount of β-globin in a transduced erythroid cell. This assumes that most of the circulating cells would be transfected, which in practice will not be the case. A value of 50% would therefore be the minimum acceptable expression level. In early studies only a 0.1–5% level of β-globin was obtained in mouse bone marrow transplantation experiments, indicating a lack of appropriate genetic control (Dzierzak *et al.*, 1988; Karlsson *et al.*, 1988; Bender *et al.*, 1989). The discovery of the globin LCR could potentially overcome this problem since it was defined by its ability to confer on a linked β-globin gene, site-of-integration independent, physiological levels of erythroid-specific gene expression which is directly proportional to transgene copy number in both transgenic mice (Grosveld *et al.*, 1987) and stably transfected tissue culture cells (Blom van Assendelft *et al.*, 1989). Unfortunately the β-globin LCR consists of five erythroid-specific DNAase1 hypersensitive sites (HS1–5) distributed over 15 kb and is therefore too large to accommodate retroviral or AAV vectors. Each HS site maps to a 200–300 bp core region that consists of a high density of binding sites for both erythroid-specific and ubiquitous transcription factors (Philipsen *et al.*, 1990; Talbot *et al.*, 1990; Pruzina *et al.*, 1991; Raguz and Grosveld, unpublished). Testing of these LCR elements individually has shown that the ability to open chromatin appears to reside within HS3, as this is the only element that can function as a single copy transgene in mice (Ellis *et al.*, 1995). HS2 and 4 function as LCRs only as multiple copies. HS1 and 5 have only very low levels of activity. These data suggest that the βLCR consists of two types of elements, firstly, the 'core' of the LCR which has the capacity to generate an open chromatin domain (HS3); secondly, the other HS sites (HS2 and 4 in particular) act as exceptionally powerful enhancer elements to boost the transcriptional potency of HS3 and hence give a full, dominant activating capacity at the physiologically required level.

We propose that this enhancement is secondary to the essential 5′ HS3 element and may be mediated by DNA looping (Ptashne, 1986) to form an LCR holocomplex. The Sp1 trans-acting factor is certainly a candidate for this role as it binds to all the HS cores (Talbot *et al.*, 1990; Philipsen *et al.*, 1990; Pruzina *et al.*, 1991) and has been shown to loop DNA (Mastrangelo *et al.*, 1991; Su *et al.*, 1991), but accessory bridging or other factors may participate in this putative loop formation. In order to form loops, it is likely that the HS core elements must be separated by spacer DNA. By forming a single LCR holocomplex from all of the HS sites, this model can account for the fact that globin genes are in competition for the LCR in a polar fashion (Hanscombe *et al.*, 1991), that the activities of the individual HS sites are additive, and that all the HS sites must be present to obtain full levels of β-globin gene expression (Fraser *et al.*, 1990). The model is also consistent with the observation that all the HS sites of the LCR are developmentally stable. All these properties are difficult to explain by models that do not invoke a holocomplex and that are based on specific HS site/promoter interactions. The concept of a holocomplex also has important implications for the molecular mechanism of gene expression and its implications for therapeutic intervention (see below).

In practical terms for viral vector development it is therefore clear which parts of the LCR would have to be used to obtain therapeutic levels of expression, but the exact size and spacing requirements of the enhancing elements are not known. We are presently testing combinations of HS3 with minimized versions of the other elements to fit existing retroviral and AAV vectors and obtain high titre virus stocks. An alternative approach using 'synthetic' vectors has also been initiated. This approach relies on the delivery of plasmid via ligand- or antibody-mediated DNA transfer and has the advantage that the size of the DNA is not limiting, i.e. it is clear which elements can be used, but the methodology to introduce such constructs into cells efficiently still has to be worked out. The real advantage of synthetic vectors is that they would be much easier to develop as drugs. Individual components, such as the DNA, the ligand or antibody, endosomal escape peptides etc. could be produced in bulk and stored easily. They would be linked in various combinations depending on the target and the disease into a particular delivery vehicle for a particular disease and obviate the need for large culture systems to produce viruses that have to be rebuilt and tested completely for each individual disease, involving very high costs.

3 Transcription modulation as a basis for drug discovery for the haemoglobinopathies

This is a completely novel (but rapidly growing) area of research, using transcription as a basis for drug discovery. In the case of the haemoglobinopathies it is known that if the fetal genes are expressed in the adult stage, the effects of thalassaemia or sickle cell anaemia are greatly ameliorated. In fact a number of compounds have been known for some time to have an effect on the γ-globin gene suppression, e.g. butyrates, hydroxyurea, azacytidine. Some of these compounds have progressed to clinical trials, but their therapeutic value appears quite limited. Thus there is a clear need for novel therapeutic compounds, and two fundamentally different approaches could be taken to obtain novel lead compounds: either a random screening approach without characterizing the proteins involved in suppression or a very defined approach after the characterization of suppressor proteins. The first approach depends on a good functional assay, since screening in patients is not an option, and the second requires a detailed knowledge of the role of individual transcription factors in the regulation of each of the genes. The next section describes our basic studies of human globin gene regulation during development using the mouse as the assay system. This allows us to study the regulation of globin gene expression at all stages of development and verifies at the same time whether the mouse can be used as a valid assay system.

When a complete human β-globin gene locus is introduced into transgenic mice the human genes are 'turned on' at the appropriate times of development, and ε and γ are expressed in the yolk sac like their mouse structural equivalents εy and βh1. ε is not expressed in the fetal liver (like εy), but the expression of the γ genes is only silenced at day 16 of development (Fig. 1; Strouboulis *et al.*, 1992). This is different from the βh1 gene which is not expressed in the fetal liver, and different from the normal pattern of expression of the γ globin genes which are normally only silenced after birth. The β-globin gene is expressed in the fetal liver, and adult stages concurrent with its murine structural equivalents βmaj and βmin. Experiments with an isolated γ gene show that this silencing is an autonomous property of the γ gene and its immediate flanking regions (Dillon and Grosveld, 1991). This suggests that the mouse can be used as a model system to study the different components of the silencing process. However the fact that the gene is silenced before the equivalent stage in humans suggests that there may be some fundamental differences between the human γ genes and its mouse equivalent (Gumucio et al., 1994) or differences in the silencing process in the two species. We therefore tested whether a mutation, normally correlated with the HPFH expression in human adults, also gives rise to an HPFH phenotype in transgenic mice. A single point mutation (Berry et al., 1992; Fig. 2) was introduced into the promoter of an otherwise normal γ gene and this gene was introduced into mice with an LCR and a β-globin gene. Analysis of the mice shows that the expression of the γ-globin gene is higher in the fetal liver relative to that of the β gene and that the expression persists into the adult (Fig. 2). Interestingly the total output of the locus has not been affected, i.e. the combined expression of the γ and the β gene is the same as from the β gene alone when in the presence of a silenced normal γ gene. This result is similar to that observed in human HPFH and shows that the mouse appears to be a valid assay system for the silencing of the γ genes. It also confirms that the globin genes compete with each other for the activation of the LCR (Hanscombe et al., 1989; Behringer et al., 1990; Enver et al., 1990). This process could be explained by a number of different mechanisms including the model that we have proposed, i.e. that the LCR forms a holocomplex (see above) which interacts directly with only one of the genes at any given time via the looping out of the intermediate DNA. If correct this would imply that large complexes of multiple proteins bound to the LCR interact with other large complexes of proteins at the promoter (and enhancers) of the genes. Such a mechanism would predict that it may be difficult to identify any particular transcription factor that is responsible for the silencing of the γ-globin genes and that it may be much more advantageous to look for potential drugs by screening rather than design.

Through a combination of placing an extra competing β gene at different positions in the complete β-globin locus (Dillon and Grosveld, unpublished) and a novel in situ hybridization protocol with intron-specific oligonucleotide probes (Wijgerde et al., 1995), we have recently obtained very strong evidence for the mechanism described above. In addition we and others have to date failed to identify a single protein factor to be responsible for the silencing process (Ronchi 1995). This would argue that the design of a good screening assay would presently be a more promising approach when compared to a rational drug design on the basis of a particular transcription factor. It is of course not excluded that a single transcription factor may be identified that will be able to alter the balance of γ vs β transcription, and a good candidate may be an EKLF (erythroid Kruppel-like factor)-related factor. EKLF was identified by Bieker (Miller and Bieker, 1993) as a protein that specifically binds to

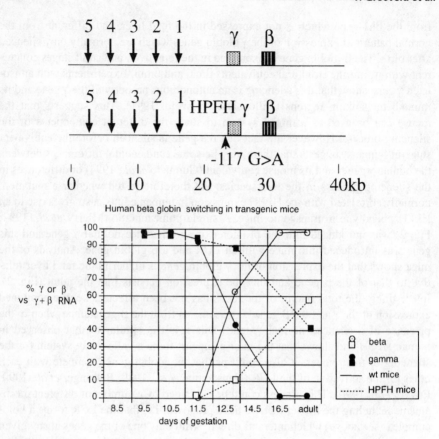

Fig. 2 Normal and HPFHγ-globin expression in transgenic mice. The top two lines show the LCR (HS1–5) coupled to a normal γ- and β-globin gene or an HPFHγ- and normal β-globin gene. The HPFH gene differs from the normal gene by a single point mutation (G>A; Berry *et al.*, 1992). The bottom panel shows the expression of these constructs when introduced into transgenic mice.

the CAC box of the β-globin promoter. The inactivation of this factor in the mouse by homologous recombination in embryonic stem (ES) cells leads to animals that fail to express the β-globin gene at appropriate levels, which results in a fatal fetal anaemia (Nuez *et al.*, 1995). We are presently determining whether the expression of the human γ-globin gene is also affected by the absence of the EKLF by crossing these mice with transgenic mice expressing the complete human β-globin locus. On the basis of homology with the mouse genes, we expect that the expression of the γ genes will not be affected which would suggest that a separate EKLF-like factor may be involved in the expression of the γ-globin gene, and that this postulated factor would be embryonic/fetal-specific in humans. If so it would provide a clear target for the development of drugs that may influence γ-globin gene expression on the basis of a particular transcription factor.

4   Screening model

The data described above suggest that at present a β-globin transgenic mouse model would be the most useful tool to screen for therapeutic drugs of potential benefit to human patients. In order to build such a model we have introduced a luciferase reporter gene at the initiation codon of the human γ-globin gene as part of an entire β-globin locus (Aγluc/loc; Fig. 3). Transgenic mice will be established and analysed at all stages of development to ensure that the still normal Gγ and the neighbouring lucAγ genes are activated early in development and silenced in the adult. They will be treated with butyrate to determine whether the genes can be reactivated in the adult.

Transgenic mice containing the Aγluc/loc will be crossed to transgenic mice containing a GATA1-T antigen construct (Cairns *et al.*, 1994) which will allow the isolation of immortalized erythroid cells in culture for further testing (see below). They will also be infected with Friend leukaemia virus to obtain murine erythroid leukaemia (MEL) cells that are genetically identical to the transgenic mice. MEL cells are erythroid cells immortalized at the proerythroblast stage and addition of DMSO, HMBA, or a number of other polar planar compounds leads to the induction of differentiation and expression of the adult mouse β-globin genes, as well as many other genes associated with terminal differentiation of erythroid cells. The two types of immortalized cells will subsequently serve as our tester cell line for novel compounds which can reactivate the human γ-globin genes. Reactivation will be monitored by using a luciferase assay which can be robotized and allows the screening of large libraries of compounds (Oncogene Science USA). Oncogene Science is

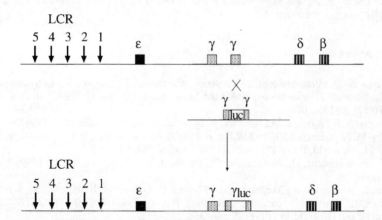

Fig. 3   The luciferase reporter locus. The top line shows the complete human β-globin locus, which is recombined with a γ-globin gene driving a luciferase reporter gene (second line) via homologous recombination. The resulting complete human β-globin reporter locus is introduced into mice by direct microinjection of the construct into fertilized mouse eggs.

currently screening a genetically engineered human erythroid cell line for activators of γ-globin gene expression. In this initial test system, the LCR enhancer HS2 and the γ-globin promoter were cloned 5′ of the luciferase reporter gene. K562 cells were transfected with the γ-globin reporter construct and stable transfectants were isolated. Individual cell clones were assayed for: (i) correct linear integration of the reporter construct; (ii) inducibility by haemin and DMSO. The chosen reporter cell line had a very good signal to noise ratio (> 100-fold) and an assay to assay coefficient of variation (CV) of < 10 % when assayed in a 96-well microtitre plate format.

To date 59 300 entities have been screened against the K562/γ-globin tester cell line in our High Throughput robotic system. These entities include both fungal extracts and purified chemicals. The percentage of entities screened resulting in a > 4-fold induction of γ-globin luciferase expression is 0.7%. Several of the active fungi extracts have been refermented and purified by bioassay guided fractionation. These activities have also shown induction of the endogenous globin levels within the tester cell line using benzidine staining for total haemoglobin levels. Further lead characterization of purified natural products and chemicals will be performed in primary erythroid cell culture systems (Fibach *et al.*, 1991) and in transgenic mice harbouring the human β-globin locus. Potential lead compounds will be tested for optimal dosage and cytotoxicity on cells in culture and then tested for their ability to activate the Gγ and lucAγ genes in the parent transgenic mouse line, thereby directly providing an animal test system before potential use in human erythroid cell cultures and in clinical trials.

Ackowledgements

This work was supported by Oncogene Science (USA), the MRC (UK), the EC and NWO (NL). N.D. was supported by the Howard Hughes Foundation, J.E. by the MRC (Canada).

References

Anagnou, N. P., Perez-Stable, C., Gelinas, R., Costantini, F., Liapaki, K., Constantopoulou, M., Kosteas, T., Moschonas, N. K. and Stamatoyannopoulos, G. (1995). *J. Biol. Chem.* **270**(17), 10256–10263.
Behringer, R. R., Ryall, T. M., Palmiter, R. D., *et al.* (1990). *Genes Devel.* **4**, 380–389.
Bender, M. A., Gelinas, R. E. and Willer, A. (1989). *Mol. Cell. Biol.* **9**, 1426–1434.
Berry, M., Grosveld, F. and Dillon, N. (1992). *Nature* **358**, 499–502.
Blom van Assendelft, G., Hanscombe, O., Grosveld, F. and Greaves, D. R. (1989). *Cell* **56**, 969–977.
Cairns, L. A., Crotta, S., Minnuzzo, M., Moroni, E, Grannucci, F., Nicolis, S., Schiro, R., Pozzi, L., Giglioni, B., Ricciardi-Castagnoli, P. *et al.* (1994). *EMBO J.* **13**, 4577–4586.
Dillon, N. and Grosveld, F. (1991). *Nature* **350**, 252–254.
Dillon, N. and Grosveld, F. (1993).*Curr. Opin. Genet. Devel.* **4**, 260–264.
Dzierzak, E., Papayannopoulou, T. and Mulligan, R. (1988). *Nature* **331**, 35–41.
Ellis, *et al.* (1995). *EMBO J.*, in press.
Enver, T., Raich, N., Ebeus, A. J. *et al.* (1990). *Nature* **344**, 309–313.

Fibach, E., Manor, D., Treves, A. and Rachmilewitz, E. A. (1991). *Int. J. Cell Cloning*, **9**, 57–64.

Fraser, P., Hurst, J., Collis, P. and Grosveld, F. (1990). *Nucl. Acid Res.* **18**, 3503–3508.

Grosveld, F., van Assendelft, G. B., Greaves, D. R. and Kollias, G. (1987). *Cell* **51**, 975.

Gumucio, D. L., Shelton, D. A., Blanchard-McQuate, K., Gray, T., Tarle, S., Heilstedt-Williamson, H., Slightom, J. L., Collins, F. and Goodman, M. (1994). *J. Biol. Chem.* **269**, 15371–15380.

Hanscombe, O., Vidal, M., Kaeda, J., Luzzatto, L., Greaves, D. R. and Grosveld, F. (1989). *Genes Devel.* **3**, 1572–1581.

Hanscombe, O., Whyatt, D., Fraser, P., Yannoutsos, N., Greaves, D., Dillon, N. and Grosveld, F. (1991). *Genes Devel.* **5**, 1387–1394.

Karlsson, S., Bodine, D., Perry, L., Papayannopoulou, T. and Nienhuis, A. (1988). *Proc. Natl. Acad. Sci.* **85**, 6062–6066.

Mastrangelo, I., Courey, A., Wall, J. *et al.* (1991). *Proc. Natl. Acad. Sci. USA* **88**, 5670–5674.

Miller, I. J. and Bieker, J. J. (1993). *J. Mol. Cell. Biol.* **13**, 2776–2786.

Nuez, B., Michalovich, D., Bygrave, A., Ploemacher, R. and Grosveld, F. (1995). *Nature*, **375**, 316–318.

Philipsen, S., Talbot, D., Fraser, P. and Grosveld, F. (1990). *EMBO J*, **9**, 2159–2167.

Pruzina, S., Hanscombe, O., Whyatt, D. *et al.* (1991). *Nucl. Acid Res.* **19**, 1413–1419.

Ptashne, M (1988). *Nature* **335**, 683–689.

Ronchi, A., Berry, M., Raguz, S., Iman, A., Yannoutsos, N., Ottlenghi, S., Grosveld, F. and Dillon, N. (1995). *EMBO J.*, in press.

Sadelain, M., Wang, C., Antoniou, W., Grosveld, F. and Mulligan, R. (1995). *Proc. Natl. Acad. Sci. USA* **92**, 6723–6732.

Strouboulis, J., Dillon, N. and Grosveld, F. (1992). *Genes Devel.* **6**, 1857.

Su, W., Jackson, S., Tijan, R. and Echols, H. (1991). *Genes Devel.* **3**, 820–826.

Talbot, D., Philipsen, S., Fraser, P. and Grosveld, F. (1990). *EMBO J.* **9**, 2169–2178.

Wijgerde, M., Grosveld, F. and Fraser, P. (1995). *Nature*, in press.

Wood, W. (1993). In *Ballière's Clinical Haematology* (D. Higgs, and D. Weatherall, eds), vol. 6, No. 1, pp. 177–213. Ballière Tindall, London.

IV

FROM TARGET TO THERAPY

9

Drug Discovery and Optimization using Binary-Encoded Small Molecule Combinatorial Libraries

JOHN C. CHABALA, JOHN J. BALDWIN,
JONATHAN J. BURBAUM, DANIEL CHELSKY,
LAWRENCE W. DILLARD, IAN HENDERSON,
GE LI, MICHAEL H. J. OHLMEYER,
TROY L. RANDLE, JOHN C. READER,
LAURA ROKOSZ and NOLAN H. SIGAL

Pharmacopeia, Inc., 101 College Road East, Princeton, NJ 08540, USA

Abstract

The mapping of the human genome continues to uncover large numbers of novel proteins, many of which may serve as the targets of drug optimization programmes for new pharmaceuticals. The rate of identification of new gene products requires new techniques that can rapidly assess and capitalize upon their therapeutic or prophylactic potential. Combinatorial chemical libraries can be utilized in two ways to help harvest the fruits of the human genome project. First, such libraries can rapidly identify molecules which bind tightly and with high selectivity to proteins, thus providing a means of elucidating the function of a given protein *in vivo*. This approach will accelerate the understanding of the role a given protein may play in disease. Secondly, combinatorial libraries can be used to enhance the rate of optimization of the properties of drug leads, thereby reducing the time required to bring a new drug to the market. An added benefit of combinatorial libraries to pharmaceutical companies is the broad patent coverage these libraries can provide.

An ideal combinatorial chemical approach would permit the rapid synthesis and bioevaluation in solution of large numbers of diverse compounds for lead identification while simultaneously supporting the rapid elucidation of the structure–function

GENOMES, MOLECULAR BIOLOGY AND DRUG DISCOVERY
ISBN 0-12-137790-3

relationships (SARs) required for optimization of drug properties. The novel binary encoding strategy employing non-sequenceable encoding molecules, the ECLiPS™ method, is described which achieves these goals. A variety of small molecule combinatorial libraries have been prepared on solid support using the ECLiPS™ technique. The library members are prepared using split synthesis employing linkers which when photolysed liberate the library members for assay free in solution. Encoding molecules which are as stable as the solid phase matrix are used in a binary code to index the reaction history of each resin particle. These molecular tags are easily attached to and selectively detached from the resin matrix. The tags are read by gas chromatography which provides a rapid and sensitive determination of the structure of each library member.

Library synthesis employs a wide variety of synthetic reactions and provides a highly diverse set of library members, especially heterocyclic compounds. The screening of two such libraries has identified lead structures for the inhibition of carbonic anhydrase (CA) as well as the outline of the SARs required for this activity. Using this information, a smaller focused combinatorial library was prepared and used to analyse the SARs governing CA inhibition and isozyme selectivity. The combination of random screening with a broad diversity of compounds followed by focused libraries for detailed SARs and selectivity demonstrates the power of binary-encoded small molecule combinatorial libraries for drug discovery and optimization.

1 Introduction

Molecular biology has provided an increasing number of new molecular targets against which pharmaceuticals may be developed for the prevention, amelioration or cure of diseases. The rapid progress made in mapping the human genome is identifying a host of additional novel proteins whose potential as pharmaceutical targets remains, in most cases, unknown. In order to determine the function of these novel proteins a variety of molecular and cell biological techniques have been employed, e.g. expression of dominant negative mutant proteins. Although molecular biological approaches are of great value in determining the function of a novel protein, the rate at which new proteins are being identified requires that other techniques be applied. Small molecules that specifically and tightly bind to a target protein have provided a valuable means of identifying and determining the function of novel proteins. Such molecules additionally often form the basis of therapy themselves, or serve as the starting point for drug optimization programmes. In most cases these small molecules were identified from natural sources, but they have also arisen from screening of synthetic compounds. Among the many examples of synthetic compounds that have served to identify new protein targets, and assisted in the elucidation of their function, are phenothiazines and synthetic adrenergic agents in the identification of G-protein-coupled receptor subtypes; acetozolamide and carbonic anhydrase; naladixic acid and bacterial gyrase; barbiturates and benzodiazepines and the GABA receptor; and verapamil and calcium channels. Although the use of small molecules to uncover protein function has been limited both by the availability of large numbers of diverse structures and by the rate at which these structures can be tested, technologies which overcome these limitations could be of enormous value.

New drugs have arisen almost exclusively from the optimization of lead compounds identified by screening of synthetic compounds and natural products. Although many pharmaceutical companies have assembled collections of synthetic compounds derived from their past drug optimization efforts, the largest of these collections contain only a few hundred thousand compounds and these collections contain only a limited diversity of structural types because they arose largely from optimization efforts of previous programmes. Compound collections of this size can be completely evaluated in modern high throughput assays within 1 year. The need for new sources of chemical diversity is particularly acute for biotechnology companies who can access large chemical collections infrequently and only at high cost. Natural products have been rich sources of structural leads that provide functional information about protein targets, and screening of materials from natural sources will continue to play an important role in lead discovery. But the rate of identification of truly novel natural structures has decreased in spite of efforts to improve screens, broaden targets, access rare organisms, and exploit unusual ecoenvironments. Although extremely valuable in lead optimization, *de novo* rational design has not uncovered lead structures. This approach is limited by the availability of crystalline or soluble targets, and the structural changes induced upon binding of small molecule inhibitors usually compromise the utility of native protein structures for molecular design. In addition, current computational models are unable to predict binding energies with sufficient precision.

Understanding the function of a novel protein and discovering a small molecule that alters protein function is only the first step in creating a new drug. A medicinal chemistry programme must nearly always be undertaken to improve the *in vitro* and *in vivo* properties of the initial lead structures which frequently suffer, for example, insufficient potency and efficacy, selectivity, or duration of action. Many lead structures possess unwanted side effects that must be eliminated, and backup compounds must be identified to replace primary candidates that frequently fail during development. The synthesis of drug analogues remains largely a manual process, and a typical medicinal chemistry optimization programme employing 10 chemists can prepare on average only a few hundred analogues per year. Hence, drug candidate optimization is both slow and expensive, frequently requiring several years at a cost of more than $5000 per analogue synthesized.

As developed over the past decade (for reviews see Gallop *et al.*, 1994; Baum, 1994; Longman, 1994), combinatorial chemistry has addressed some of the needs for more diverse chemical structures for screening, but generally has not expedited drug optimization. Combinatorial chemistry has been applied largely to the preparation of libraries of natural oligomers (Gordon *et al.*, 1994; Zuckermann *et al.*, 1994), and more recently to a small set of unnatural oligomers (Simon *et al.*, 1992; Cho *et al.*, 1993), because the synthesis of oligomers employs but a few well-studied reactions and the structures of oligomers can be elucidated using only the minute quantities of drug typically produced. Although oligomeric libraries can be extremely large (10^6–10^9 compounds), they are intrinsically limited in their structural diversity. Furthermore, when composed of natural oligomers such as peptides and oligonucleotides, a difficult optimization effort is frequently required to overcome limiting *in vivo* properties such as low oral bioavailability, short serum half-life, and poor cell penetration.

Several strategies have been employed to provide large numbers of non-sequenceable compounds without requiring their direct structure determination. Large chemical libraries have been prepared and assayed as mixtures of > 10^4 members, and active members are then identified by laborious deconvolution strategies employing selective resynthesis and reassay (Houghten *et al.*, 1991, 1992; Pinilla *et al.*, 1992). Combinatorial chemical libraries have also been prepared using spatial indexing to encode the reaction history and predicted structure at fixed synthetic sites (Geysen *et al.*, 1984, 1968; Fodor *et al.*, 1991; Geysen and Mason 1993; Jacobs and Fodor 1994). However, assaying large libraries using spatial indexing has required that the product remain attached to the solid support, thereby creating the possibility for spurious results induced by the presence of the support and limiting the testing of such libraries to certain types of biochemical assays. In an attempt to overcome these shortcomings, encoding strategies employing co-synthesis of microsequenceable oligonucleotides (Brenner and Lerner, 1992; Needels *et al.*, 1992) or peptides (Kerr *et al.*, 1993; Nikolaiev *et al.*, 1993) have been developed. Microsequenceable encoding introduces additional problems, however, such as cumbersome and time-consuming chemical protection and deprotection, as well as limitations on the variety of chemical reactions which can be employed to prepare individual library members. In addition, the decoding of the structure of library members using peptide microsequencing or polymerase chain reaction (PCR) amplification of DNA limits the rate at which structure–function data can be accumulated from high throughput screening.

2 Overview of binary-encoded combinatorial library synthesis

The binary-encoded combinatorial libraries synthesis approach (ECLiPS™, first described by Ohlmeyer *et al.* (1993) and developed at Pharmacopeia, Inc.) permits the preparation of very large libraries of small molecules for random screening as well as smaller focused libraries built around active structures for elucidation of SARs (Burbaum *et al.*, 1995). ECLiPS™ marries split synthesis of combinatorial libraries on resin supports, first described by Furka and co-workers (Furka *et al.*, 1988a,b, 1991; Sebestyen *et al.*, 1993), also known as 'portion-mixing' (Lam *et al.*, 1991) or 'divide couple and recombine' (Houghten *et al.*, 1991) with a robust encoding technology employing highly stable tags that identify the synthetic steps a given resin bead has experienced. The tags form a binary molecular 'bar code' that is easily, rapidly and reliably attached, detached and read.

A schematic representation of binary-encoded combinatorial synthesis is provided in Fig. 1. A functionalized resin support is divided among several reaction vessels and a different reaction is performed in each flask. Upon completion and workup of each reaction, a unique set of tags is attached directly to the resin which encodes the reaction performed in each vessel. The resin batches in each flask are then pooled, reapportioned into several flasks, and the next cycle of synthesis and unique tagging is performed. The process of division, reaction, tagging and pooling is repeated until the desired combinatorial library is produced wherein each member is uniquely encoded. In the simplest case the total number of compounds produced is found by multiplying the number of subdivisions in each step. For example, if four steps were employed using subdivisions into 10, 15, 20 and 25 reaction flasks, the total number of compounds produced would be $10 \times 15 \times 20 \times 25 = 75\,000$. As illustrated in Fig. 1, each encoding molecule is independently attached to the support and used as a bit in a binary code. The two key advantages of using tags in a binary format are: (i) only the presence or absence of a given tag needs to be determined, obviating the need for microsequencing, and (ii) a small number of tags can encode a very large combinatorial library since the number of encodable molecules is given by 2^n (where n is the number of tags). Although as many as 40 tags can easily be prepared, permitting the encryption of $2^{40} = $ ca $1\,000\,000\,000\,000$ library members, only 15–18 tags are required to encode libraries of several hundred thousand members.

The tags (Fig. 2) are simple haloaryloxyalkanols whose trimethylsilyl ethers are easily separated by gas chromatography and detectable at femtomolar levels by electron capture (ECGC; Ohlmeyer *et al.*, 1994). The tags are attached directly to the resin matrix using a carbene insertion reaction (Nestler *et al.*, 1994) which does not significantly affect the bound drug, as evidenced by analysis of products prepared and tagged in bulk (Baldwin *et al.*, personal communication, 1994). Because tag detection is so sensitive, the total mass of tags attached to a given resin particle is only a few per cent of the mass of the encoded structure.

The tags and their linking groups are as stable as the resin itself and therefore do not impose any additional constraints on the chemical reaction conditions compatible with solid phase synthesis. Indeed, the number and kinds of synthetic reactions that can be successfully performed on solid support is growing exponentially, and already includes not only extensions of known acylation and phosphorylation chemistries, but also a wide variety of heteroatomic bond-forming reactions (e.g. acetal and ketal formation, sulfonylation; *N*-, *O*- and *S*-alkylation, *N*-heteroalkylation, and reductive amination), as well as a number of key carbon–carbon bond-forming reactions, including aldol condensations, Diels–Alder reactions, 1,3-dipolar addition, Suzuki reactions, Stille couplings and Wittig reactions.

Once an interesting bioactivity is associated with a given bead, the tags are selectively detached using ceric ammonium nitrate oxidation and silylated prior to ECGC (Fig. 3). The oxidative detachment requires about 1 h and is conveniently performed in parallel in arrays of microreaction vessels. Analysis of tag sets to identify a structure requires less than 15 min each, and using autoinjection one ECGC instrument can easily read 50 or more structures each day. The rapid structural prediction of hundreds of compounds is a key advantage of the ECLiPS™ technology.

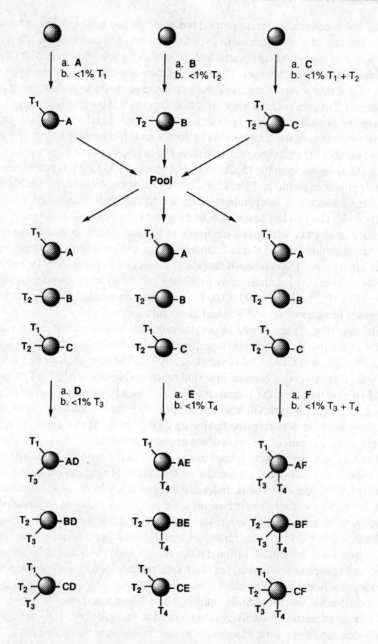

Fig. 1 Schematic representation of binary-encoded combinatorial synthesis. (Reprinted with permission from Chabala, J. C., Baldwin, J. J., Burbaum, J. J. *et al.* (1994) *Perspect. Drug Discov. Design* **2**, 305. Copyright 1995, Escom Science Publishers B.v.)

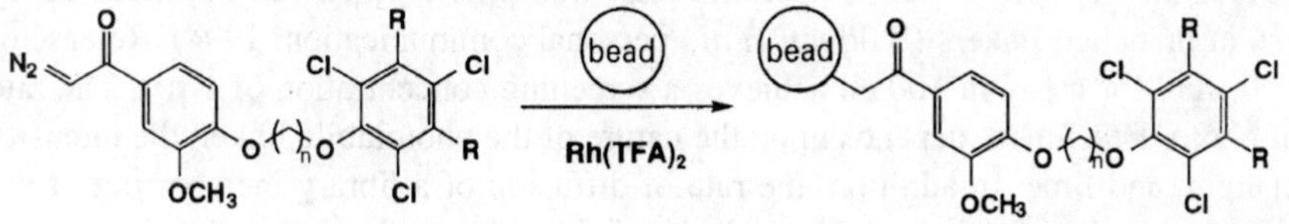

R = H, n = 3–12
and
R = Cl, n = 4–6 (linear library)
R = Cl, n = 5, 6 (heterocyclic library)

Fig. 2 Attachment of encoding molecules using $Rh(TFA)_2$-catalysed carbene insertion. (Reprinted with permission from Chabala, J. C., Baldwin, J. J., Burbaum, J. J. *et al.* (1994) *Perspect. Drug Discov. Design* **2**, 305. Copyright 1995, Escom Science Publishers B.v.)

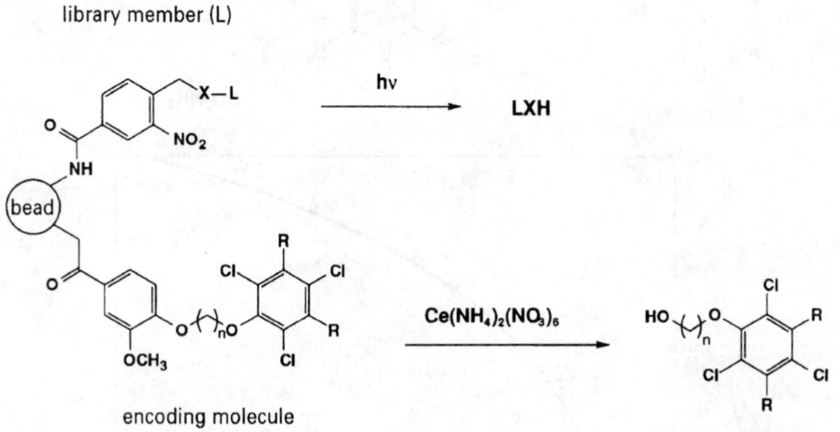

R = H, n = 3–12
and
R = Cl, n = 4–6 (linear library)
R = Cl, n = 5, 6 (heterocyclic library)

Fig. 3 Orthogonal detachment of library members and tags. Library members are released for assay in solution by photolysis. The tags encoding the structure of the active compound are released oxidatively. (Reprinted with permission from Chabala, J. C., Baldwin, J. J., Burbaum, J. J. *et al.* (1994) *Perspect. Drug Discov. Design* **2**, 305. Copyright 1995, Escom Science Publishers B.v.)

The library members are attached to the solid support through a photolabile *o*-nitrobenzyl linkage which permits the rapid and predictable release of compound (Fig. 3) for assay in solution without the introduction of additional reagents which may compromise biological assessment. Photolytic detachment can be partial or complete, and by measuring photolysis rates of specific linkers, known quantities of ligand can be semiquantitatively detached. The total achievable loading of a given compound on an unmodified 130 μm diameter Tentagel™ (Rapp Polymere,

Tübingen, Germany) bead is approximately 300 pmol, which can be increased by use of branched linkers (Baldwin *et al.*, personal communication, 1994). Release of 100 pmol for assay in 100 ml achieves a screening concentration of 1 μM. The rate of photo-detachment depends upon the nature of the photolabile linker, the intensity of light, and time. In addition, the rate of diffusion of a library member out of the bead into bulk solvent must be considered. In order to determine the appropriate photo-elution conditions for a given library, several members of varying physical properties are prepared in bulk in a non-combinatorial fashion, and their photo-elution and bead diffusion characteristics determined. The result of a typical photo-elution experiment (compound **3**, below) is shown in Fig. 4. Since little

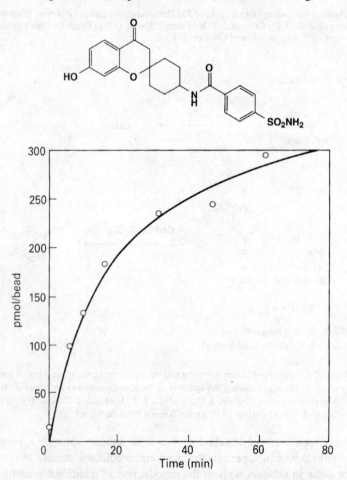

Fig. 4 Photo-elution of PC931370 (**3**). Sealed vials each containing 20 beads carrying **3** suspended in 100 ml of acetonitrile were photo-eluted at 365 nm at ambient temperature for the times shown. The points represent averages of three determinations. (Reprinted with permission from Chabala, J. C., Baldwin, J. J., Burbaum, J. J. *et al.* (1994) *Perspect. Drug Discov. Design* **2**, 305. Copyright 1995, Escom Science Publishers B.v.)

variation in photolysis rate is observed as a function of linker, it is assumed that the detachment of other library members does not vary greatly. Solvent contact times are optimized for the slowest observed diffusion rates.

A two-step arraying and photo-elution process is employed for the biological assay of large libraries. Several beads (typically 10–20) are placed in each well of a 96-well microtitre plate (master plate), a portion of the compound on each bead is photo-eluted, and the products are transferred by filtration to a daughter plate. After evaporation of the solvent, the dry products are then available for resolubilization in bioassay media. When an active well is identified in a daughter plate, the corresponding beads in the master plate are rearrayed singly, and additional compound is photo-eluted, transferred, and reassayed to identify the single bead responsible for the observed activity. Analysis of the tags on the bead which carried the active molecule provides the structure of the active compound. Using this approach, assaying a 1 000 000-member library arrayed at 30 beads per well requires about 350 96-well plates, a number easily handled by current high-throughput formats.

3 Combinatorial library synthesis and structure encoding

The ECLiPS™ binary encoding technology has been used to prepare several heterocyclic and other small molecule (Henderson *et al.*, 1994) libraries. The generic structures and some representative members of two such libraries, a linear and a heterocyclic library, respectively, are shown in Figs 5 and 6. Both libraries were designed so that a few per cent of their members bore an aromatic sulfonamide, a group known to bind to the zinc of CA and inhibit enzymatic activity, and screening of these libraries was therefore expected to uncover compounds active against CA. Although incorporation of commercially available synthons could have easily permitted the synthesis of libraries with over 30 000 members, the libraries were intentionally kept small (6727 and 1143 members, respectively) to permit rapid screening of multiple copies of the library. When screened in this way, active structures were decoded multiple times, thus providing evidence for fidelity of their synthesis.

The linear library was synthesized in three combinatorial steps employing seven synthons in the first step, and 31 synthons in each of the second and third steps. In the first step four *N*-Fmoc (9-fluorenylmethoxycarbonyl)-protected amino alcohols and three *N*-Fmoc protected amino acids were coupled to aminofunctionalized Tentagel™ via a photocleavable *o*-nitrobenzyl linker. Amino acids were attached directly to linker-modified resin by esterification, while amino alcohols were first coupled through carbonates to the linkers which were then coupled to resin by amide formation. Each of the seven resin batches was then tagged using unique combinations of three of the tags shown in Fig. 2. The seven resin batches were pooled, deprotected, and divided into 31 lots. Each lot was coupled via amide bond formation with one of 31 Fmoc-protected amino acids. Each of the lots was tagged, pooled, deprotected, and again divided into 31 lots. Each lot was allowed to react with one of a variety of 31 functionalized sulfonyl chlorides, isocyanates, carboxylic acids and chloroformates to provide

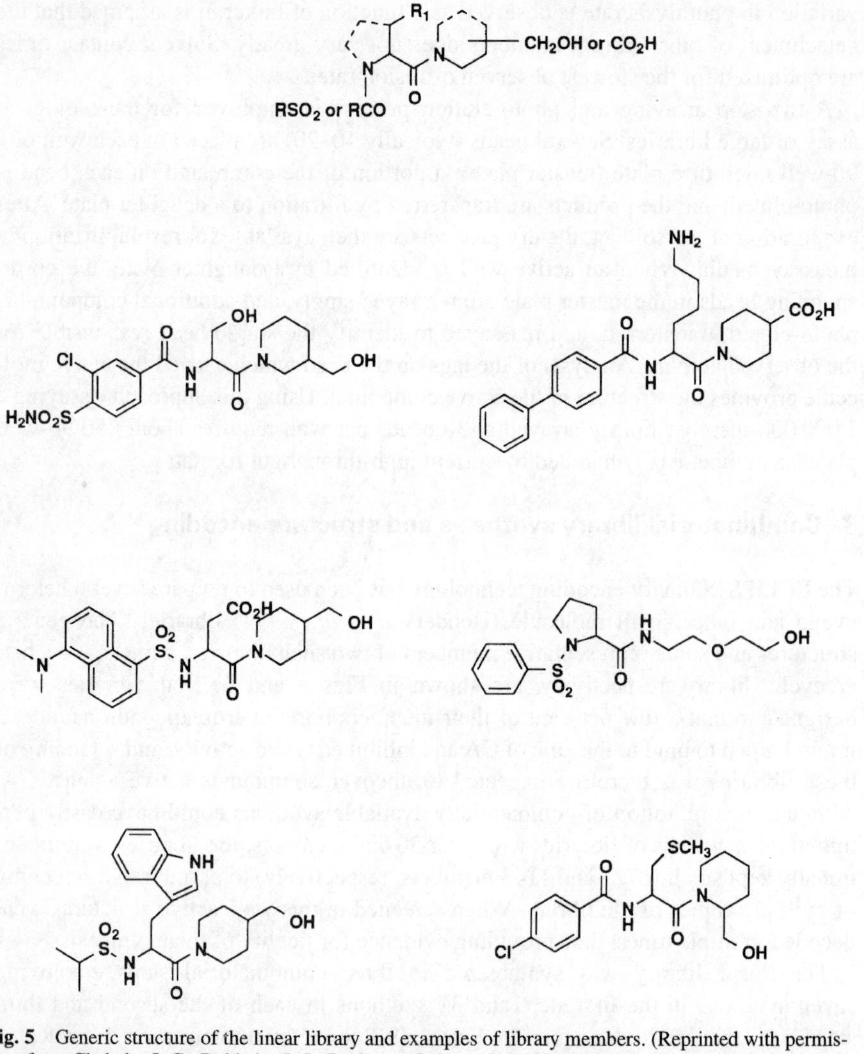

Fig. 5 Generic structure of the linear library and examples of library members. (Reprinted with permission from Chabala, J. C., Baldwin, J. J., Burbaum, J. J. *et al.* (1994) *Perspect. Drug Discov. Design* **2**, 305. Copyright 1995, Escom Science Publishers B.v.)

sulfonamides, ureas, amides and carbamates. After tagging and pooling, the completed library contained 6727 members.

The heterocyclic library was prepared in a more complex manner (Fig. 7) which illustrates the flexibility of the ECLiPS™ approach. Three dihydroxyacetophenones were coupled to the photo-cleavable linker, and the products were then attached through amide linkages to three batches of amino functionalized Tentagel™. After tagging, the resin batches were pooled, divided into seven portions, and condensed with seven ketones to form dihydrobenzopyrans (Batch A). Three resin batches

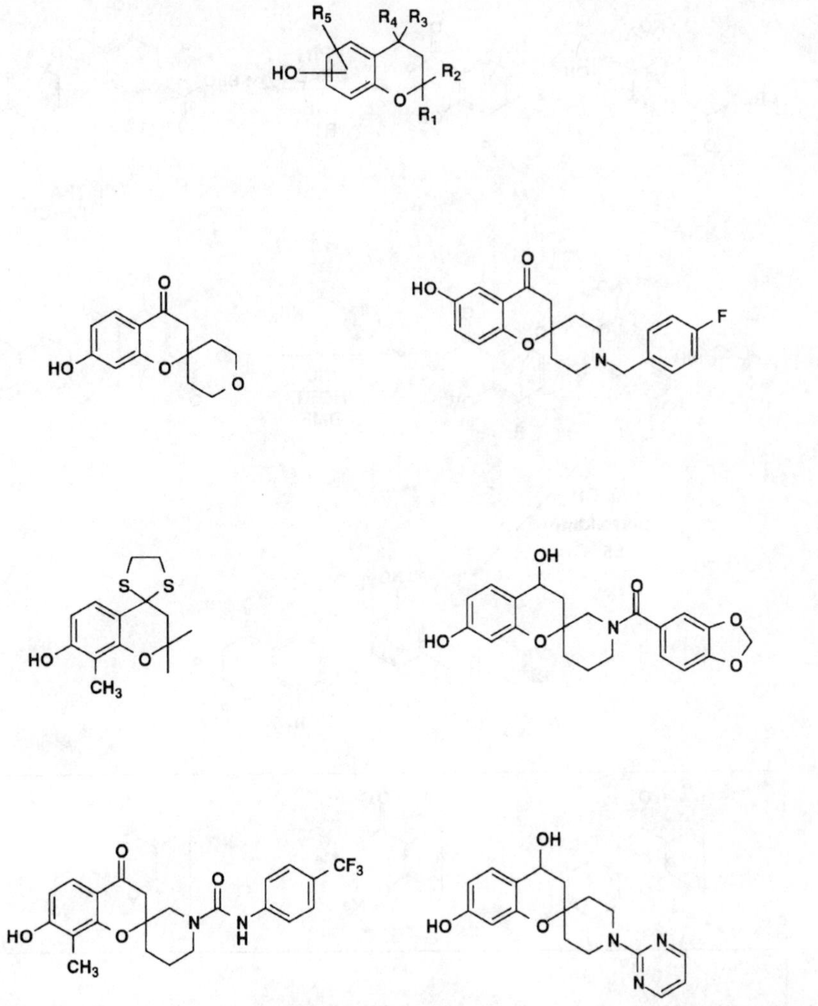

Fig. 6 Generic structure of the heterocyclic library and examples of library members. (Reprinted with permission from Chabala, J. C., Baldwin, J. J., Burbaum, J. J. *et al.* (1994) *Perspect. Drug Discov. Design* **2**, 305. Copyright 1995, Escom Science Publishers B.v.)

which did not contain Boc (*t*-butyloxycarbonyl)-protected amines (Batch B) were separated, and the four remaining resin batches bearing *N*-Boc groups were separately pooled, deprotected and neutralized (Batch C). Batch C was divided into 41 lots, 30 of which were used to form amides, ureas, carbamates, thioureas and sulfonamides. These 30 portions were then tagged and mixed (Batch D). In addition, 10 of the remaining lots of Batch C were used for reductive alkylation with a set of six aldehydes and heteroaromatic displacement with a set of four chloroheterocycles to

Fig. 7

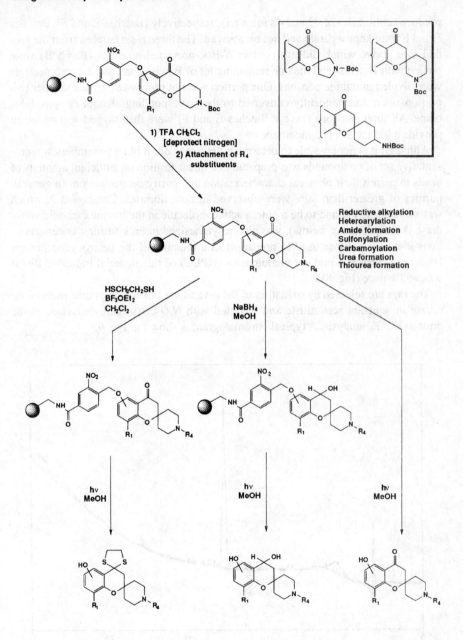

Fig. 7 Schematic flow chart for the synthesis of the benzopyran library. (Reprinted with permission from Chabala, J. C., Baldwin, J. J., Burbaum, J. J. *et al.* (1994) *Perspect. Drug Discov. Design* **2**, 305. Copyright 1995, Escom Science Publishers B.v.)

produce sublibraries of 72 and 48 members, respectively (Batches E and F). Batches E and F were kept separate and not bioassayed. The three resin batches from the second step above which did not contain *N*-Boc-protected products (Batch B) were pooled with Batch D and the one remaining lot of Batch C, and these combined lots were divided into three portions. One portion was not processed, while the other two portions were independently converted to the corresponding alcohol or spirodithiolane. All three portions (except Batches E and F) were then tagged and mixed to provide a library of 1143 members.

Although it is not possible to determine the purity of all library members, a representative set of compounds was prepared in a linear fashion on sufficient amounts of beads to permit their physical characterization and purity determination. In general, purities of greater than 80% were observed in both libraries. Compound **3**, which was subsequently found to be a potent active molecule in the bovine carbonic anhydrase II (bCAII assay, below), was also resynthesized in bulk fashion under conditions identical to those used to prepare it as a member of the heterocyclic library. High performance liquid chromatography (HPLC) of this material indicated that it was >95% pure (Fig. 8).

The tags are released by oxidation of the *o*-vanillate linker using ceric ammonium nitrate in aqueous acetonitrile and silylated with *N,O*-bis(trimethylsilyl)acetamide prior to ECGC analysis. A typical chromatogram is shown in Fig. 9.

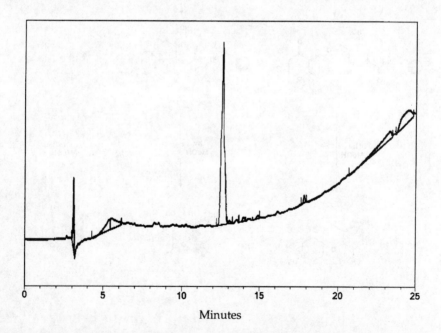

Minutes

Fig. 8   A reverse phase HPLC chromatogram of crude PC931370 (**3**) prepared on solid phase and photoeluted as in Fig. 4. (Reprinted with permission from Chabala, J. C., Baldwin, J. J., Burbaum, J. J. *et al.* (1994) *Perspect. Drug Discov. Design* **2**, 305. Copyright 1995, Escom Science Publishers B.v.)

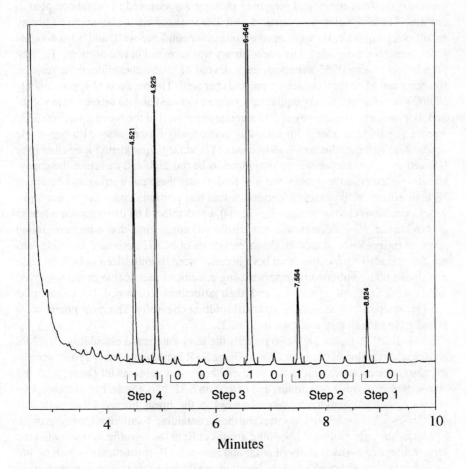

Fig. 9 A representative ECGC chromatogram and the structure it encodes. (Reprinted with permission from Chabala, J. C., Baldwin, J. J., Burbaum, J. J. *et al*. (1994) *Perspect. Drug Discov. Design* **2**, 305. Copyright 1995, Escom Science Publishers B.v.)

4 Lead discovery and optimization

The linear and the heterocyclic libraries were screened against bovine CA isozyme II (bCAII) using a fluorescence-based dansylamide displacement assay (Ponticello *et al.*, 1987; Burbaum *et al.*, 1995). Resin beads from each library were distributed in 96-well microtitre plates, library members were photo-eluted using 365 nm irradiation, and free compounds were filtered into daughter plates which were then dried. When assayed at 10 compounds per well approximately 1.4% of the heterocyclic library and 6% of the linear library exhibited activity (the libraries contained 3% and 10% of arylsulfonamides, respectively). Because the hit rates were so high, the initial multiple compound screening strategy was changed to single compounds per well. The photo-eluted products of over 2300 beads from the heterocyclic library (two library equivalents) were assayed one compound per well, and 33 individual active beads were decoded. The linear library was screened in two portions. The first portion, containing 3255 members, each devoid of a benzenesulfonamide residue, was screened as mixtures of ten compounds per well. The products of approximately 17 000 beads (ca five library equivalents) were evaluated and no actives were identified. Because an initial survey at 10 compounds per well of the second portion (3472 members) exhibited a high hit rate, this portion was further assayed using single beads. Assay of the eluates of 4608 beads (1.3 library equivalents) identified over 600 actives. This hit rate was again judged to be too high and therefore the dansylamide concentration was increased 600-fold. Under these more stringent conditions 18 high affinity actives were identified within this portion. Under the higher stringency conditions chlorothiazide (K_D ~75 nM) was displaced by dansylamide whereas acetazolamide (K_D ~7.5 nM) was not displaced, suggesting that structures found active in the presence of increased concentrations of bCAII possessed K_D values <75 nM. Several active structures from both libraries were resynthesized in bulk on resin in a linear, non-combinatorial manner using conditions identical to those employed during combinatorial synthesis, and their structures confirmed by comparison against materials prepared using standard solution chemistry. The most potent compound from each library is shown in Table 1.

The ECLiPS™ technology also permits the semi-automated elucidation of SARs and the optimization of drug candidates. Using SAR hypotheses derived from screening a large library, more structurally focused libraries are subsequently being prepared whose members are chosen to test and extend an SAR hypothesis. For example, two classes of active compounds were observed in the linear library, those with 2,4-dichloro-5-sulfamoylphenyl moieties and those containing 4-sulfamoylphenyl groups. The latter strongly preferred lipophilic groups at R_2 in the L-configuration, while the former tolerated a wide variety of polar and non-polar R_2 substituents in both D- and L-configurations. Although 4-chloro-3-sulfamoylphenyl-substituted compounds were included in this library, no such structures were uncovered upon screening. Independent synthesis and bioassay of compound **2** confirms that its potency was above the detection limits under the more stringent assay conditions. Observations of this type validate the use of this screening approach to selectively detect potent compounds and

Table 1 Structures 1–3 were confirmed using ^{1}H-NMR spectroscopy and mass spectrometry. (Reprinted with permission from Chabala, J. C., Baldwin, J. J., Burbaum, J. J. *et al.* (1994) *Perspect. Drug Discov. Design* **2**, 305. Copyright 1995, Escom Science Publishers B.v.)

Compound	Number	K_d bCAII (nM)
	1	4
	2	660
	3	15

also support synthesis and bioassay of binary tag-encoded combinatorial libraries as a means to identify divergent SARs.

The ECLiPS™ approach can also be utilized to achieve selective biological activity. A focused sublibrary of 217 members was prepared based upon the most potent bCAII inhibitor **1**. In this library the 4-sulfamoylphenyl moiety was held constant while the R_1 and R_2 substituents were systematically varied by incorporation of natural and unnatural amino acids (Fig. 10). In these experiments, the library members were completely photo-eluted from the resin support, divided equally, and assayed against bCAII and human carbonic anhydrase I (hCAI). The results are plotted in Fig. 10 (Chelsky, 1993, 1994). As expected, most of the compounds were quite active but non-selective, falling on the 45° diagonal. A few compounds which exhibited >50% inhibition of dansylamide binding fell on or near the axes, and therefore appeared to exhibit selective inhibition of a particular enzyme (larger points in

Fig. 10). This experiment was repeated several times, and the same apparently selective structures were decoded repetitively, suggesting that approximately equivalent quantities of ligand were photo-eluted from different beads. The combinatorial synthesis of the focused library, its biological evaluation, and the resynthesis and confirmation of activity of active compounds required the activities of two chemists and one biologist over an approximately 2 month period. These results illustrate the potential of binary-encoded combinatorial synthesis to elucidate SAR information and to rapidly identify compounds with desirable selectivity properties.

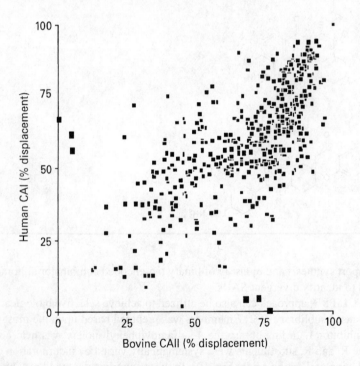

Fig. 10 Selectivity plot of the arylsulphonamide sublibrary against human carbonic anhydrase I and bovine carbonic anhydrase II. For this experiment compounds were completely detached from the solid support by photolysis in methanol, the solutions were divided into two equal aliquots, and tested against hCAI and bCAII. The percentage of dansylamide displaced by the test compound was calculated by assigning a value of 100 to the least fluorescent well, and a value of 0 to the most fluorescent well, then normalizing the remaining data vs these two extremes. (Reprinted with permission from Chabala, J. C., Baldwin, J. J., Burbaum, J. J. *et al.* (1994) *Perspect. Drug Discov. Design* **2**, 305. Copyright 1995, Escom Science Publishers B.v.)

Acknowledgements

The authors would like to thank Dr Gregory L. Kirk, Joseph Brezinski, Peter Kieselbach, and Nicole White of the Department of Bioengineering of Pharmacopeia, Inc., who provided valuable technical assistance in the manipulation and decoding of the combinatorial libraries.

References

Baum, R. M. (1994). *Chem. Eng. News* February 7, 20.

Brenner, S. and Lerner, R. A. (1992). *Proc. Natl. Acad. Sci. USA.* **89**, 5381.

Burbaum, J. J., Ohlmeyer, M. H. J., Reader, J. C., Henderson, I., Dillard, L. W., Li, G., Randle, T. L., Sigal, N. H., Chelsky, D. and Baldwin, J. J. (1995). *Proc. Natl. Acad. Sci. USA* (in press).

Chabala, J. C., Baldwin, J. J., Burbaum, J. J., Chelsky, D., Dillard, L. W., Henderson, I., Li, G., Ohlmeyer, M. H. J., Randle, T. L., Reader, J. C., Rokosz, L. and Sigal, N. H. (1994). *Perspect. Drug Discov. Design* **2**, 305.

Chelsky, D. (1993). 1st Int. Conf. on Advanced Pharmaceutical Substance Screening. Vienna, Austria, 29 November – 2 December.

Chelsky, D. (1994). 1994 Int. Forum on Adv. in Screening Methodologies. Princeton, NJ, 17–20 April.

Cho, C. Y., Moran, E. J., Cherry, S. R., Stephans, J. C., Fodor, S. P. A., Adams, C. L., Sundaram, A., Jacobs, J. W. and Schultz, P. G. (1993). *Science* **261**, 1303.

Fodor, S. P. A., Read, J. L., Pirrung, M. C., Stryer, L., Lu, A. T. and Sols, D. (1991). *Science* **251**, 767.

Furka, A., Sebestyen, F., Asgedom, M. and Dibo, G. (1988a). In *Abstr. 14th Int. Congr. Biochem.* (Prague, Czechoslovakia) vol. 5, p. 47.

Furka, A., Sebestyen, F., Asgedom, M. and Dibo, G. (1988b). In *Abstr. 10th Int. Symp. Med. Chem.* (Budapest, Hungary), p. 288.

Furka, A., Sebestyen, F., Asgedom, M. and Dibo, G. (1991). *Int. J. Pept. Protein Res.* **37**, 487.

Gallop, M. A., Barret, R. W., Dower, W. J., Fodor, S. P. A. and Gordon, E. M. (1994). *J. Med. Chem.* **37**, 1233.

Geysen, H. M. and Mason, T. J. (1993). *Bioorg. Med. Chem. Lett.* **3**, 397.

Geysen, H. M., Meloen, R. H. and Barteling, S. J. (1984). *Proc. Natl. Acad. Sci. USA* **81**, 3998.

Geysen, H. M., Rodda, S. J. and Mason, T. J. (1986). *Mol. Immunol.* **23**, 709.

Gordon, E. M., Barrett, R. W., Dower, W. J., Fodor, S. P. A. and Gallop, M. A. (1994). *J. Med. Chem.* **37**, 1385.

Henderson, I., Ohlmeyer, M. and Baldwin, J. J. (1994). 2nd Annual Cambridge Healthtech Institute Development of Small Molecule Mimetic Drugs. Philadelphia, PA, 11–12 April.

Houghten, R. A., Pinilla, C., Blondelle, S. E., Appel, J. R., Dooley, C. T. and Cuervo, J. H. (1991). *Nature* **354**, 84.

Houghten, R. A., Appel, J. R., Blondelle, S. E., Cuervo, J. H., Dooley, C. T. and Pinilla, C. (1992). *BioTechniques* **13**, 412.

Jacobs, J. W. and Fodor, S. P. A. (1994). *Trends Biotechnol.* **12**, 19.

Kerr, J. M., Banville, S. C. and Zuckermann, R. N. (1993). *J. Am. Chem. Soc.* **115**, 2529.

Lam, K. S., Salmon, S. E., Hersh, E. M., Hruby, V. J., Kazmierski, W. M. and Knapp, R. J. (1991). *Nature* **354**, 82.

Longman, R. (1994). *In Vivo,* **12**, 23.

Needels, M. N., Jones, D. G., Tate, E. H., Heinkel, G. L., Kochersperger, L. M., Dower, W. J., Barrett, R. W. and Gallop, M. A. (1992). *Proc. Natl. Acad. Sci. USA.* **90**, 10700.

Nestler, H. P., Bartlett, P. A. and Still, W. C. (1994). *J. Org. Chem.* **59**, 4723.

Nikolaiev, V., Stierandova, A., Krchnak, V., Seligmann, B., Lam, K. S., Salmon, S. E. and Lebl, M. (1993). *Pept. Res.* **6**, 161.

Ohlmeyer, M. H. J., Swanson, R. N., Dillard, L. W., Reader, J. C., Asouline, G., Kobayashi, R., Wigler, M. and Still, W. C. (1993). *Proc. Natl. Acad. Sci. USA* **90**, 10922.

Ohlmeyer, M., Henderson, I., Burbaum, J., Swanson, R., Chelsky, D. and Baldwin, J. J. (1994). 2nd Annual Cambridge Healthtech Institute Development of Small Molecule Mimetic Drugs. Philadelphia, PA, 11–12 April.

Pinilla, C., Appel, J. R., Blanc, P. and Houghten, R. A. (1992). *BioTechniques* **13**, 901.

Ponticello, G. S., Freedman, M. B., Habecker, C. N., Lyle, P. A., Schwam, H., Varga, S. L., Christy, M. E., Randall, W. C. and Baldwin, J. J. (1987). *J. Med. Chem.* **30**, 591.

Sebestyen, F., Dibo, G., Kovacs, A. and Furka, A. (1993). *Bioorg. Med. Chem. Lett.* **3**, 413.

Simon, R. J., Kania, R. S., Zuckermann, R. N., Huebner, V. D., Jewell, D. A., Banville, S., Ng, S., Wang, L., Rosenberg, S., Marlowe, C. K., Spellmeyer, D. C., Tan, R., Frankel, A. D., Santi, D.V., Cohen, F. E. and Bartlett, P. A. (1992). *Proc. Natl. Acad. Sci. USA* **89**, 9367.

Zuckermann, R. N., Martin, E. J., Spellmeyer, D. C., Stauber, G. B., Shoemaker, K. R., Kerr, J. M., Figliozzi, G. M., Goff, D. A., Siani, M. A., Simon, R. J., Banville, S. C., Brown, E. G., Wang, L., Richter, L. S. and Moos, W. H. (1994). *J. Med. Chem.* **37**, 2678.

10

Monoclonal Antibodies: Tools for Exploiting Gene Discovery

DAVID P. BLOXHAM

Celltech Therapeutics Ltd, 216 Bath Road, Slough SL1 4EN, UK

Abstract

During the last few years there has been a dramatic increase in the discovery of new genes encoding proteins with extracellular domains such as novel cytokines, adhesion molecules and cell surface proteins (e.g. receptors). Generally these molecules participate in complex biological interactions between macromolecules, and the design of synthetic antagonists to block their effect for therapeutic purposes is frequently extremely difficult if not impossible. In contrast to synthetic antagonists it is relatively straightforward to produce a mouse monoclonal antibody as a functional antagonist of a human protein and given the extracellular location of these proteins they are accessible to antibodies both *in vitro* and *in vivo*. By a process of genetic engineering a mouse antibody can be converted to a novel human antibody. These humanized antibodies, characterized by high potency, exquisite selectivity, long half-life, low immunoreactivity and good safety, make ideal reagents to validate the therapeutic concept either in animal models or human disease. This approach will be illustrated by considering results with antibodies to TNFα, CD18 and IL-5 showing how their use in animal models can guide therapeutic strategy. Moreover, recent studies in humans with a recombinant antibody to TNFα, CDP571, have shown such encouraging results in active rheumatoid arthritis that it may well prove to be a useful drug in its own right.

1 Introduction

The principal challenge in pharmaceutical research is the selection of the correct target to produce the desired therapeutic effect. Today this problem is growing ever more complex. Progress in gene sequencing technology suggests that within the foreseeable future all the genes which are expressed on the human genome will be identified. The number of genes is expected to be of the order of 80 000–100 000.

GENOMES, MOLECULAR BIOLOGY AND DRUG DISCOVERY
ISBN 0-12-137790-3

Clearly, not all these genes will be linked to human disease. Nevertheless, given the inventiveness of the human mind it would not be unreasonable to anticipate that 1–10% of these new genes would be potential targets for therapeutic intervention. Assuming that pharmaceutical companies set out to pursue all these targets then this would be a prodigious effort in terms of human resource and total research and development expenditure. These costs have to be set against the changing environment of cost containment in the provision of health care. For the pharmaceutical companies this has led to an ever greater desire that their own research programmes should be innovative, executed rapidly and have a clearer probability of success. The most successful companies of the future will be those that are the most effective in selecting the correct therapeutic target. This chapter will discuss this process of target selection and, hopefully, prove that the use of therapeutic antibodies could be a key component of a company's armamentarium of approaches in achieving some of the objectives outlined above.

2 Principles of target selection

The main approaches to validating a therapeutic target are as follows:

(i) Knock out a specific gene in an animal model system to prevent the onset or induction of a disease process.
(ii) Over-express a target gene to produce the effects of the disease process.
(iii) Use selective antagonists of a target gene product to block the disease process.

Nowadays there are many elegant examples of the first two approaches. Common examples of gene knock-outs are found in human or rodent diseases. For example, cystic fibrosis can be attributed to a specific gene defect resulting in defective chloride ion transport (Harris, 1992). Clearly, restoring chloride transport across epithelia will be a major therapeutic goal in the treatment of cystic fibrosis. In an alternative example, tumour cells frequently carry mutations in the transcription factor, p53 (Donehower et al., 1992). Transfection of normal p53 into cancer cells, an example of over-expression, restores normal control of cell growth and indicates that this would be a valid target for therapeutic intervention (Yin et al., 1992).

The fundamental problem with the first two approaches is that the information that they produce is most readily exploited by gene therapy companies. Furthermore, many human diseases have a polygenic susceptibility. Gene knock-out experiments can be very useful in giving information on what the therapeutic and toxicological effects of a gene product inhibitor are likely to be. Unfortunately, they are of little help in identifying the inhibitor. This brings us to the third approach, using specific antagonists.

Traditionally, pharmaceutical companies have validated therapeutic approaches by using synthetic molecules either to antagonize receptor–ligand interactions or to inhibit enzymes. These new chemical entities are easily tested in animal models and if effective they are readily exploited in the treatment of human diseases. Indeed this approach has been the basis of the dramatic success of the pharmaceutical industry over the past century. At its most successful the approach has led to the rational design and discovery of the vast majority of modern medicines. This synthetic approach works best when the ligand for a receptor or the substrate of an enzyme has a relatively small molecular weight. However, the progress of molecular biology has provided a wealth of examples of macromolecular interactions which are key messengers in biological systems. For example, there is considerable effort in most large pharmaceutical companies to develop novel treatments for autoimmune diseases based on the advances in our understanding of the immune system. However, virtually every messenger (the cytokines) in the immune system is a protein with a molecular weight in excess of 10 000. The molecules which trigger the migration of cells in the immune system (the adhesion molecules) are also complex glycoproteins of high molecular weight.

Using first principles it is virtually impossible to design effective antagonists of these processes which have sufficient binding information to be effective. However, antagonists of these proteins are readily available using monoclonal antibody technology. Monoclonal antibodies provide ideal reagents for validating a therapeutic target and in certain circumstances they may also provide first generation therapeutic reagents which can be used clinically.

3 Properties of antibodies which can be exploited for therapeutic purposes

The main advantage of antibodies is that they bind to molecules of a wide range of molecular weights with very high affinity (10^{-9}–10^{-12}M) and virtually total selectivity. Antibodies can be produced easily which bind to cytokines, adhesion molecules or ligand receptors. Their specificity is such that it is usually quite straightforward to distinguish between proteins which have highly conserved amino acid sequences but which have different spatial epitopes. Indeed, before gene sequencing became routine as a means of classifying different protein products, antibodies were commonly used in distinguishing between different but related biological activities.

A further feature of antibodies is that their properties are dependent on the epitope that they recognize. Thus, in interacting with a receptor, antibodies can bind in such a way that they block the active site, thus acting as a functional antagonist. Alternatively they can bind to the receptor in a manner which mimics the natural ligand and trigger activation of the receptor.

A further feature of antibodies which can be exploited therapeutically is that once they have bound to their ligand, the constant regions of the antibody within the immune complex can trigger both complement-mediated lysis and cellular cytotoxicity. Thus, if the ligand is expressed upon the surface of a cell (e.g. CD4 and CD8 on T-cells) the binding to specific antibodies can be used selectively to deplete cell populations carrying the relevant marker. Thus, anti-CD4 antibodies can be used to selectively deplete helper T-cells and anti-CD8 antibodies can be used for suppresser T-cells (Newman *et al.*, 1992). The possible range of uses of a family of antibodies in modifying a ligand–receptor interaction is shown in Fig. 1.

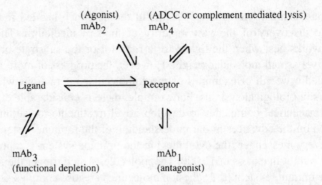

Fig. 1   Uses of monoclonal antibodies in modifying ligand–receptor interactions.

The final advantage of antibodies is that, provided they do not provoke an immune reaction, once in the circulation they have very long residence times with elimination half-lives that may be as long as a month (Hakimi *et al.*, 1991). This means that in principle a single administration of an antibody will give long-term therapeutic cover. Everyone who has been involved in drug discovery will have endured the frustration of trying to find synthetic molecules with satisfactory drug metabolism and pharmacokinetic properties to evaluate whether a target pharmacological effect can be achieved in an animal model. This can be especially difficult if the compound is to be used in a chronic model which takes weeks for an effect to develop. With antibodies this problem does not exist. Generally it is sufficient to determine the half-life in the chosen species (which will usually be in days) and then design a therapeutic dosing schedule which maintains the antibody above the concentration required.

4   Genetic engineering has revolutionized the potential for antibody use *in vivo*

The discovery by Kohler and Milstein (1975) of the technique for monoclonal antibody production has had a profound effect on all areas of biology in the past 20 years and has revolutionized much of diagnostic medicine. Nevertheless, their impact on therapeutic medicine has been minimal and until this year the only therapeutic monoclonal antibody in clinical use was the OKT3 antibody for the prevention of transplant rejection. The reason for this is that until recently the only available monoclonal antibodies were primarily derived from rodent sources. These rodent monoclonal antibodies provoke such a profound immune response in human and non-human primates that their use is restricted to single dose acute therapies. Clearly, if antibodies are to be used more widely then this immunogenicity problem has to be solved. Recent progress in molecular biology appears to have overcome this difficulty (Mountain and Adair, 1992).

The structure of antibodies of the IgG class can be broken down into three component parts. Thus, the carboxyl domains of the heavy and light chains are reasonably constant depending on the antibody isotype. The antigen binding sequences are located at the amino terminal variable regions of the heavy and light chains and comprise six linear sequences (three on each chain) known as the complementarity determining regions (cdr). These cdr sequences are supported by the framework regions of the variable domain. Using primers targeted at these conserved sequences it has become relatively straightforward to clone the variable regions of heavy and light chains using polymerase chain reaction (PCR) technology (Jones and Bendig, 1991). By selecting appropriate combinations of the cdr sequences, the framework regions and the constant regions, it is possible to create artificial antibodies (Winter and Milstein, 1991).

If the cdr regions of a mouse antibody are transplanted into human acceptor framework and constant regions then this will create a novel human antibody which in principle should be virtually indistinguishable from a natural human antibody. Clearly this should eliminate the immunogenicity associated with murine antibodies and allow the antibody to be used in human and non-human primates.

The original technique for cdr grafting developed by Winter and his colleagues (Jones *et al.*, 1986) does not always permit the full recovery of antigen binding activity due to unfavourable interactions between residues in the cdr sequence and the framework region. However, with greater experience in this area it has proved possible to identify the most important framework residues and appropriate compensatory changes of these amino acids nearly always leads to full recovery of binding affinity (Adair *et al.*, 1994).

During the past few years the approach to humanizing antibodies has been supplemented with a number of alternative stratagems to produce human antibodies. For example, human antibodies can be cloned directly from patients who have been exposed to antigens (Burton *et al.*, 1991). This approach could be readily applied to isolate human antibodies cross-reacting with infectious organisms. This is particularly powerful when linked to the process of repertoire cloning and display of fused heavy and light chain variable sequences linked to surface proteins on filamentous phage (McCafferty *et al.*, 1990). Antibodies recognizing a specific antigen can then be selected by the process of panning for phage followed by rounds of phage replication to amplify the target sequence. In principle, the affinity of an antibody isolated in this manner can be further enhanced by rounds of *in vitro* mutagenesis (Glaser *et al.*, 1992).

Human antibodies can also be isolated by more complex procedures of molecular biology. For example, the SCID mouse has been reconstituted with part of the human immunoglobulin gene repertoire. When this mouse is immunized with an antigen it naturally produces a novel human antibody (Duchosal *et al.*, 1992).

5 Specific problems associated with antibody use

The creation of novel human antibodies may have solved the immunogenicity problem in humans but unfortunately it does create a new set of problems when these antibodies are used in animal models. Firstly, antigen recognition by antibodies is so specific that frequently antigen recognition does not cross species barriers, i.e. an anti-human antigen antibody will not recognize the same antigen from a rodent species. If this proves to be the case then it will be obligatory to use a primate disease model to evaluate the efficacy of the antibody. Alternatively, if a transgenic model exists that functionally expresses the human target protein then this would be an ideal model. As an example, there is a transgenic mouse that abnormally expresses human tumour necrosis factor α (TNFα) and develops signs of a polyarthritis at 3–4 weeks after birth. If this mouse is treated with anti-human TNFα the polyarthritis is prevented (Keffer *et al.*, 1991). This clearly implicates TNFα in the pathology of rheumatoid arthritis and suggests that an anti-TNFα antibody could be effective in treatment of the disease.

A second problem with novel human antibodies is that they are profoundly immunogenic in rodents and this limits their ability to be used in toxicology or animal models. This can be overcome by a further round of genetic engineering in which the novel human antibody is converted to a human–rodent chimeric antibody by replacing the constant regions with the appropriate rodent sequences. Although chimeric antibodies are still somewhat immunogenic, they are clearly superior to antibodies with a complete species mismatch (Lo Buglio *et al.*, 1989).

Some of the challenges associated with antibody use are generic and independent of the species source of the antibody. Firstly, antibodies have high molecular weight and this means that there is little possibility of delivering antibodies by the oral route. Rather, it seems almost certain that antibodies will have to be delivered by injection.

A more significant problem is that the high molecular weight will limit the penetration of the antibody. The most accessible targets will be those where the antigen is present in the vascular space. Alternatively, antibodies may gain access to the extravascular space in circumstances where there is a breakdown in local permeability barriers. For example, inflammation causes an enhanced permeability of the synovial membrane which enhances the access of therapeutic antibodies to the synovial space.

Finally, it should always be borne in mind that the biosynthesis of a monoclonal antibody is a complex biological process and the cost of their production is going to remain relatively high in comparison to new chemical entities for the foreseeable future. Therefore it is critically important that in selecting an antibody as a therapeutic agent the antibody should possess a property that is not easily duplicated by a synthetic molecule.

Despite the problems which have been highlighted in this section, on balance the unique properties of antibodies and the breakthrough in reducing the problems of immunogenicity associated with immunoglobulins means that there has been an enormous growth in their development as novel therapeutic entities. I shall highlight some developments that are ongoing for their use in the treatment of septic shock, rheumatoid arthritis and asthma.

6 Septic shock

Despite the advances in the development of powerful antibiotics, septic shock remains a significant and increasing clinical problem (Glauser *et al.,* 1991). Currently there are nearly 500 000 cases of septic shock annually and this number continues to increase due to the increase in the number of immuno-suppressed individuals and the use of progressively more complex surgical procedures in cardiac and gastrointestinal surgery.

Septic shock is normally triggered by an occluded infection and is characterized by a profound fall in blood pressure, a change in core body temperature and progressive failure of normal tissue perfusion. Although the response is initiated by infectious organisms, particularly Gram-negative bacteria, it has become clear that most of the adverse effects are produced as a consequence of over-reaction of the host to the infectious insult. The problem is how to block over-reactive processes of the host rather than to destroy the infectious organism.

Infection triggers the activation of macrophages and increases the production of a number of cytokines including TNFα. TNFα is a pleiotropic hormone which has a number of actions which could be directly responsible for the syndrome of septic shock (Beutler and Cerami, 1989) . For example TNFα has direct effects on the cardiovascular system causing vasodilatation which could be responsible for the dramatic fall of blood pressure observed in shock. Furthermore, TNFα induces the up-regulation of the expression of adhesion molecules, particularly in the lungs. The expression of these adhesion molecules (E-selectin; β2 integrins such as lymphocyte function associated molecule-1 (LFA1), Mac 1 (also known as integrin CR3) and p150,95 (Springer, 1990)) plays a key role in the accumulation of inflammatory cells (e.g. neutrophils, macrophages) which are important in the elimination of the infectious organism. In the case where the infection is occluded and not easily resolved by the inflammatory cells, then their over-accumulation will lead to tissue damage.

It should be possible to block the inflammatory cascade at a large number of points to prevent septic shock. Initially we were interested in comparing whether it would be preferable to block the effects induced by TNFα or to block the function of adhesion molecules. In order to decide between these two approaches we chose to compare the effects of an anti-TNF antibody and an anti-CD18 antibody (CD18 is a conserved protein component of the integrin adhesion molecules) in a baboon model of septic shock. In this model, adult baboons are treated with the appropriate antibody or saline followed by an *Escherichia coli* challenge which results in death and significant organ damage within 72 h.

Progressively increasing the anti-TNF dose completely prevented mortality (see Table 1) and significantly reduced the damage to organs. In contrast, anti-CD18 actually increased mortality and resulted in greater organ pathology. Clearly this result indicates that blockade of TNF is a more appropriate therapeutic goal in the treatment of septic shock when compared to blockade of integrin function. It is not clear why anti-CD18 should exacerbate the model but it seems most probable that the accumulation of inflammatory cells in an integrin-dependent manner is essential

Table 1 Therapeutic effects of antibodies in a baboon septic shock model

	Alive	Dead	% 72 h survival	Organ pathology
Control	1	7	13	+++
Anti-TNF (0.1 mg kg^{-1})	4	2	67	++
Anti-TNF (1 mg kg^{-1})	6	0	100	+/−
Anti-CD18 (1 mg kg^{-1})	0	5	0	++++

for resolution of the infection. Enhancing susceptibility to infection would be an obvious concern for any long-term use of a CD18 antagonist.

Although the results with anti-TNF in septic shock models in animals have been most encouraging, it has proved much more difficult to demonstrate this therapeutic benefit in human clinical studies.

The most extensive clinical study with an anti-TNF antibody has been conducted by Bayer using the murine antibody, BAY X 1351 for the treatment of sepsis and septic shock. This Phase III study, Norasept 1, was carried out at 31 centres in North America and involved treatment with placebo or two doses of drug (7.5 or 15 mg kg^{-1}) to patients who were receiving current best patient management in an intensive care unit. Initially, sepsis all comers (both shock and non-shock) were recruited to the trial but an interim analysis showed that there was no therapeutic benefit in the group without shock (shock was defined as a sustained fall in blood pressure below 90 mmHg systolic). In total, 330 non-shock sepsis patients were treated with BAY X 1351 during the trial and there was no evidence for any adverse effects on mortality.

In the final phase of the trial only septic shock patients were recruited. In all, 971 patients were treated of whom 478 (49%) were in shock (Wherry *et al.,* 1993). There was a numerical reduction of 17.3% in overall mortality in the shock group at 28 days after treatment although this reduction did not reach statistical significance. There was no detectable difference in the two treatment doses. Most strikingly, treatment with BAY X 1351 resulted in almost 50% reduction in acute mortality at the early time points in the study (e.g. at 3 days). The interpretation of this data is that treatment with the anti-TNF may save the life of individuals who would have died of septic shock (dying acutely) against a background of continuing mortality in other individuals due to the underlying disease which precipitated the septic shock.

More recently, Bayer has presented the results of a second septic shock study (Intersept 1) in 553 patients treated with 3 and 15 mg kg^{-1}. This study showed a statistically significant reduction in the duration of shock which is consistent with the animal model results. Again there was a numerical reduction in the incidence of mortality but this did not achieve statistical significance.

It has been estimated that the size of treatment groups would have to be increased about six-fold in order to achieve statistical significance at a reasonable statistical power. As a consequence of this, Bayer is conducting a 1900 patient septic shock trial. This trial commenced at the beginning of 1994 and involves two treatment groups, i.e. placebo and 7.5 mg kg^{-1} BAY X 1351. The results are expected in 1996.

7 Rheumatoid arthritis

Rheumatoid arthritis is a chronic autoimmune disease characterized by both local inflammatory destruction of articular cartilage and bone, leading to joint destruction and systemic inflammation. In the joint there is a characteristic proliferation of synovial cells and an infiltration of inflammatory cells. TNF levels in synovial fluid are consistently elevated in rheumatoid arthritis patients. The known actions of TNF could contribute to the pathogenesis of rheumatoid arthritis in a number of ways. For example, TNF stimulates collagenase production by synovial cells which could be directly involved in the degradation of the cartilage (Dayer et al., 1985). TNF also stimulates proliferation of synovial cells.

One of the first questions that can be asked is whether a direct antagonist of TNF will be effective in arthritis or whether it is necessary to deplete all the TNF-producing cells. In order to address this problem, two chimeric antibodies were created starting from the hamster anti-rodent TNF antibody, TN3 (Sheehan et al., 1989). In the first, the constant regions were replaced by the murine γ2a sequences to create a complement-fixing antibody capable of neutralizing murine TNF and depleting cells expressing TNF on their surface. In the second chimeric antibody, the murine γ1 non-complement-fixing sequence was used creating an antibody which is effectively a pure TNF antagonist (Suitters et al., 1994).

These two antibodies have been tested in a murine model of arthritis induced by the administration of type II collagen. The antibodies were administered either prior to the collagen (prophylactic treatment) or once the arthritis symptoms had developed (therapeutic treatment). The γ1 chimeric antibody was active when administered in both the prophylactic and therapeutic dosing regimens suggesting that TNF neutralization alone was sufficient to achieve efficacy. The γ2a chimeric antibody was similarly active in both dosing regimens. This antibody did appear to be superior at longer times (greater than 40 days) after administration in the prophylactic mode. This result could be attributed either to a longer half-life of the antibody in the circulation or to the depletion of memory T-cells which recognize type II collagen and express the membrane-bound form of TNF on their cell surface.

The evidence that a TNF antagonist is effective in animal models of arthritis provides a clear incentive for all medicinal chemists trying to achieve this objective with a synthetic molecule that either prevents the biosynthesis of TNF or directly antagonizes its action. This approach has been reinforced further by results which are appearing from human clinical trials in rheumatoid arthritis patients. There are now two antibodies that have been successfully evaluated in rheumatoid arthritis patients. cA2 is a chimeric antibody, developed by Centocor

160   D. P. Bloxham

(Elliott *et al.*, 1993), capable of complement fixation (human γ1 isotype) and
CDP571 is a novel human antibody, developed by Celltech (Stephens *et al.*,
1994), which does not fix complement (human γ4 isotype). Both antibodies have
been evaluated in patients with active rheumatoid arthritis who have previously
failed existing drug therapy in placebo-controlled double-blind studies. The results
from both trials were most encouraging (Elliott *et al.*, 1994a; Rankin *et al.*, 1995).
Both antibodies cause statistically significant improvements in subjective (pain,
joint swelling, tender joints) and quantitative (acute phase reactants such as C-
reactive protein) disease parameters. What was particularly encouraging was that
both antibodies produced significant responses within 2 weeks of treatment, which
is in marked contrast to results with other treatments such as methotrexate where
much longer periods (e.g. 12 weeks) are required to demonstrate benefit. Indeed,
quite a number of patients treated with the antibodies reported a rapid onset of a
feeling of well-being and a diminution in the lethargy which is commonly associated with rheumatoid arthritis.

The initial results of multiple administration with both antibodies were also
encouraging. In repeated therapy with the monoclonal antibody cA2, seven patients
who completed two to four cycles of treatment (Elliot *et al.*, 1994b) showed good
repeated clinical response in both swollen joint count and C-reactive protein. Four
of the patients did develop human anti-chimeric antibodies (HACAs) which seemed
to result in a reduction in the response duration in later cycles of treatment. In contrast to the results with the chimeric antibody, the novel human antibody CDP571
appears to have been better tolerated on multiple administration. Figure 2 shows the
pharmacokinetic profile following the administration of CDP571 on four occasions

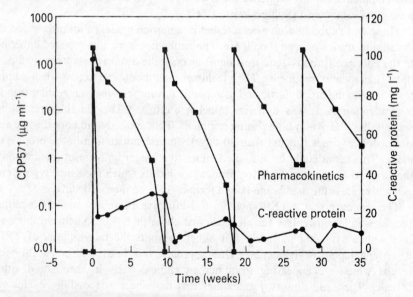

Fig. 2 Multiple administration of CDP571 to rheumatoid arthritis patients, 4×10 mg kg^{-1}.

to a rheumatoid arthritis patient. Multiple administration over 8 months did not affect the pharmacokinetic profile of the drug. Furthermore, the plasma concentration of C-reactive protein, a marker of inflammation, after an initial fall on drug treatment, was maintained within the levels expected for a normal individual (10–20 mg l^{-1}). Our measurements of the immune response to CDP571 in humans indicate that the titre of the immune response is very low and actually decreases further as the dose of CDP571 is increased, suggesting that individuals are tolerized to the novel human antibody. Clearly, if this is the case then it bodes well for the long-term potential for treatment with an anti-TNF antibody. Furthermore, it should be recognized that the adverse events associated with both cA2 and CDP571 are not very significant. This has to be set against the background that most current treatments for rheumatoid arthritis, particularly disease modifying anti-rheumatoid drugs, are associated with very significant toxicity. It now remains to establish that the therapeutic effects of the anti-TNF antibodies can be maintained in Phase III clinical trials. If they can, then there is every possibility that this new modality will represent a breakthrough therapy in rheumatoid arthritis. Furthermore, it is possible that those agents will be active in inflammatory bowel diseases, such as Crohn's disease and ulcerative colitis, as well as other autoimmune diseases such as multiple sclerosis and diabetes.

8 Asthma

Eosinophils are one of the most abundant cell types infiltrating into the lungs of asthmatics and they have been implicated in the damage associated with pulmonary inflammation (Durham and Kay, 1985). Interleukin-5 (IL-5) is a selective eosinophil effector in humans that enhances eosinophil production and release from bone marrow, chemotaxis, activation and survival (Yamaguchi et al., 1988). Antagonism of IL-5 could be a novel approach to controlling inflammation and airway hyperreactivity without causing the generalized immunosuppression that is commonly found with oral steroid therapy.

Today, asthma is usually managed either with an inhaled β_2-agonist bronchodilator or anti-inflammatory drug (steroids, chromoglycate). These products are used by the inhalation route because their side effects preclude systemic administration. We were interested in evaluating whether an anti-IL-5 antibody could be an effective therapy with different efficacy and an improved safety profile. However, we were keenly aware that an antibody would be an expensive product and if it was to be successfully used then additional advantages would have to be found. In particular, we have concentrated upon the duration of therapeutic effect as a key parameter. Initially we had expected to see a long duration of action in primates consistent with the slow clearance of antibodies from the circulation. However, as will become clear, these studies show an interesting feature which, if duplicated in asthma, could influence our approach to novel therapy in this area.

Initially, the effect of an anti-IL-5 antibody on an antigen challenge (Ascaris) in cynomolgus monkeys was evaluated (Egan et al., 1995). Essentially monkeys were treated with antibody followed by aerosol antigen challenge and some 24 h later the accumulation of eosinophils was measured as well as the dose of histamine required to produce a 40% decrease in dynamic compliance of the airways. This showed that the antibody at a dose of $0.3\,mg\,kg^{-1}$ caused a profound inhibition of both the eosinophilia in the lungs as well as blocking the hyperreactivity to histamine aerosol. What was particularly interesting about this experiment was revealed when the time to recover the sensitivity to *Ascaris* challenge was followed. This showed that 3 months after antibody challenge the *Ascaris* response was completely blocked even though the antibody had been eliminated from the circulation. Eventually the *Ascaris* response was recovered at 6 months post-antibody treatment. Clearly this result raises the possibility that antibodies might produce prolonged therapeutic responses. How this effect is achieved is quite unknown. It does open a novel therapeutic prospect for the anti-IL-5 antibody because it could be administered to asthmatic patients prior to the allergen season. In this situation the antibody might have a protective effect throughout the season and prevent the complications that are frequently observed in asthma patients due to elevated allergens in the air they breathe. This concept remains to be demonstrated in human asthmatics. As a result of a collaboration between Schering-Plough and Celltech, a novel human anti-IL-5 antibody, SCH55700, is in the process of being evaluated for its therapeutic efficacy in asthma.

9 Conclusions

The use of therapeutic antibodies has not made much clinical impact during the past decade. The principal reason for this is that antibodies were only readily available using the original hybridoma technology of Milstein and Kohler. Progress in genetic engineering has changed this picture completely and it is now reasonably straightforward to custom design an antibody for virtually any purpose involving their use as antagonists, agonists or to deplete cell populations. In this way antibodies have proved to be an invaluable tool in probing the validity of a particular therapeutic approach. What has become more clear recently is that novel human antibodies are plausible candidates for use in human therapy and there is now a burgeoning interest in using antibodies in a wide range of applications. 1995 saw the first approval by the FDA of ReoPro™, a human–mouse chimeric anti-GPIIbIIIa antibody, as the first representative of this new class of genetically engineered antibody, in this case for use in high risk patients undergoing angioplasty. It is also anticipated that the anti-IL-2 receptor antibody developed by Roche and Protein Design Laboratories will be submitted for regulatory approval for the treatment of graft versus host disease in transplant rejection. Clearly, it is hoped that these singular events mark the dawn of a new era in therapeutic medicine when all the evolutionary information contained in the genetic information encoding antibodies is finally unlocked. At the very least, antibodies offer a new class of product with a selective interaction which no synthetic drug has ever achieved and this, it is hoped, will translate to enhanced safety of these new products.

Acknowledgements

I am indebted to numerous colleagues at Celltech, Bayer and Schering-Plough for giving me access to the results presented in this review. I am particularly grateful to Mark Bodmer, Roly Foulkes, Martyn Robinson, Sue Stephens and Mark Sopwith, all of Celltech, for their help in preparing this manuscript.

References

Adair, J. R., Athwal, D. S., Bodmer, M. W., Bright, S. M., Collins, A. M., Pulito, V. L., Rao, P. E., Reedman, R., Rothermel, A. L., Xu, D., Zivin, R. A. and Joliffe, L. K. (1994). *Hum. Antibod. Hybridomas* **5**, 41–47.

Beutler, B. and Cerami, A. (1989). *Annu. Rev. Immunol.* **7**, 625–655.

Burton, D. R., Barbas, C. F., Persson, M. A. A., Koenig, S., Chanock, R. M. and Lerner, R. A. (1991). *Proc. Natl. Acad. Sci. USA* **88**, 10134–10137.

Dayer, J. M., Beutler, B. and Cerami, A. (1985). *J. Exp. Med.* **162**, 2163–2168.

Donehower, L. A., Harvey, M., Slagle, B. L., McArthur, M. J., Montgomery, C. A., Butel, J. S. and Bradley, A. (1992). *Nature* **356**, 215–221.

Duchosal, M. A., Eming, S. A., Fischer, P., Leturq, D., Barbas, C. F., McConahey, P. J., Caothien, R. H., Thornton, G. B., Dixon, F. J. and Burton, D.R. (1992). *Nature* **355**, 258–262.

Durham, S. R. and Kay, A. B. (1985). *Clin. Allergy* **15**, 411–418.

Egan, R. W., Atwahl, D., Chou, C., Emtage, S., Jehn, C., Kung, T. T., Mauser, P. J., Murgolo, N. J. and Bodmer, M. W. (1995). *Int. Arch. Allergy Immunol.*, in press.

Elliott, M. J., Maini, R. N., Feldman, M., Long-Fox, A., Charles, P., Katsikis, P., Brennan, F. M., Walker, J., Bijl, H., Ghrayeb, J. and Woody, J.N. (1993). *Arthr. Rheum.* **36**, 1681–1690.

Elliott, M. J., Maini, R. N., Feldman, M., Kalden, J. R., Antoni, C., Smolen, J. S., Leeb, B., Breedveld, F. C., MacFarlane, J. D., Bijl, H. and Woody, J. N. (1994a). *Lancet* **344**, 1105–1110.

Elliott, M. J., Maini, R. N., Feldman, M., Long-Fox, A., Charles, P., Bijl, H. and Woody, J. N. (1994b). *Lancet* **344**, 1125–1127.

Glaser, S. M., Yelton, D. E. and Huse, W. D. (1992). *J. Immunol.* **149**, 3903–3913.

Glauser, M. P., Zanetti, G., Baumgartner, J. D. and Cohen, J. (1991). *Lancet* **338**, 732–739.

Hakimi, J., Chizzonite, R., Luke, D. R., Familletti, P. C., Bailon, P., Kondas, J. A., Pilson, R. S., Lin, P., Weber, D. V., Spence, C., Mondini, L. J., Tsien, W., Levin, J. L., Gallati, V. H., Korn, L., Waldmann, T. A., Queen, C. and Benjamin, W. (1991). *J. Immunol.* **147**, 1352–1359.

Harris, A. (1992). *Br. Med. Bull.* **48**, 738–753.

Jones, T. S. and Bendig, M. M. (1991). *Biotechnology* **9**, 88–89.

Jones, P. T., Dear, P. H., Foote, J., Neuberger, M. S. and Winter, G. (1986). *Nature* **321**, 522–525.

Keffer, J., Probert, L., Cazlaris, H., Georgopoulos, S., Kaslaris, E., Kioussis, D. and Kollias, G. (1991). *EMBO J.* **10**, 4025–4031.

Kohler, G. and Milstein, C. (1975). *Nature* **265**, 495–497.

Lo Buglio, A. F., Wheeler, R. H., Trang, J., Haynes, A., Rogers, K., Harvey, E. B., Sun, L., Ghrayeb, J. and Khazaeli, M. B. (1989). *Proc. Natl. Acad. Sci. USA* **86**, 4220–4224.

McCafferty, J., Griffiths, A. D., Winter, G. and Chiswell, D. J. (1990). *Nature* **348**, 552–554.

Mountain, A. and Adair, J.R. (1992). *Biotechnol. Genet. Eng. Rev.* **10**, 1–142.

Newman, R., Alberts, J., Anderson, D., Carner, K., Heard, C., Norton, F., Raab, R., Reff, M., Shuey, S. and Hanna, N. (1992). *Biotechnology* **10**, 1455–1460.

Rankin, E. C. C., Choy, E. H. S., Kassimos, D., Kingsley, G. H., Sopwith, A. M., Isenberg, D. A. and Panayi, G. S. (1995). *Br. J. Rheumatol,* in press.

Sheehan, K. C. F., Ruddle, N. H. and Schreiber, R. D. (1989). *J. Immunol.* **142**, 3884–3893.

Springer, T. A. (1990). *Nature* **346**, 425–433.

Stephens, S., Emtage, S., Vetterlein, O., Athwal, D., Chaplin, L., Sopwith, M. and Bodmer, M.W. (1994). *J. Cell Biochem.* Suppl. 18D, 216.

Suitters, A. J., Foulkes, R., Opal, S. M., Palady, J. E., Emtage, J. S., Rolfe, M., Stephens, S., Morgan, A., Holt, A. R., Chaplin, L. C., Shaw, N. E., Nesbitt, A. M. and Bodmer, M. W. (1994). *J. Exp. Med.* **179**, 849–856.

Wherry, J., Wenzel, R., Wunderlink, R., Silverman, H., Perl, T., Nasraway, S., Levy, H., Bone, R., Balk, R. and Allred, R. (1993). *33rd Interscience Conference on Antimicrobial Agents and Chemotherapy*, Abstract 696.

Winter, G. and Milstein, C. (1991). *Nature* **349**, 293–299.

Yamaguchi, Y., Suda, T., Suda, J., Eguchi, M., Miura, Y., Harad, N., Taminaga, A. and Takatsu, K. (1988). *J. Exp. Med.* **167**, 43–56.

Yin, Y., Tainsky, M. A., Bischoff, S. Z., Strong, L. C. and Wahl, G. M. (1992). *Cell* **70**, 937–948.

11

Retroviral Vectors: First-Generation Systems for Gene Therapy

DAVID E. ONIONS

Department of Veterinary Pathology, University of Glasgow, The Veterinary School, Glasgow G61 1QH, UK

Abstract

A key element of gene therapy is the requirement to introduce a therapeutic gene into the correct cells and promote the expression of that gene for an extended period. Introducing genes into cells can be accomplished efficiently in the laboratory but the techniques are not generally appropriate for clinical application. Viruses must enter living cells in order to replicate, so increasing attention has been paid to using genetically modified viruses as vehicles for gene therapy.

Viruses from several different families, particularly adenovirus and adeno-associated viruses, have been developed as vectors. Amongst the most useful vectors are those derived from retroviruses, a family which includes HIV and cancer-causing viruses of several animal species. Of the first 70 gene therapy applications approved in the USA over 60 involved the use of retrovirus vectors. Vectors based on subgroups of murine and feline leukaemia viruses appear to be particularly promising as these viruses are very efficient at infecting human cells, a property that is in part determined by their envelope glycoprotein spikes which bind to receptors on human cells. During the life cycle of these viruses the RNA genome of the virus is reverse transcribed into a DNA provirus and integrated into chromosomal DNA. It is this feature that makes retroviruses attractive tools for gene therapy, for once a provirus is integrated into a stem cell all of the progeny cells will inherit a copy of the vector sequences.

Retrovirus vectors are not without their disadvantages. The oncogenicity of their parental viruses is related to their capacity to activate oncogenes at their sites of insertion and vectors require modification to reduce this risk. Secondly they are limited in the size of insert they can deliver and by the titres of vectors that can be achieved.

As gene therapy becomes more sophisticated there is a need to develop targeting

GENOMES, MOLECULAR BIOLOGY AND DRUG DISCOVERY
ISBN 0-12-137790-3

vectors, particularly if disseminated cancer is to be tackled. Targeting involves two complementary approaches: first, modification of the receptors on viruses, and second the incorporation of tissue-specific regulatory elements so that the transcription of the gene of interest is controlled. Progress in both areas is going to depend on advances in several areas, particularly the tissue-specific regulation of transcription.

For all of these virus vectors the design of safe systems and rigorous laboratory testing of their safety is of paramount consideration. In the future we may expect to see safer, hybrid systems which exploit viral proteins or protein motifs to assist synthetic vectors to enter cells and avoid degradation of their vector DNA. Whatever vectors come into widespread use, a fundamental understanding of the biology of viruses will have played an important part in their evolution.

1 Introduction

The central paradigm of gene therapy is the introduction of genetic information into a specific population of cells followed by the appropriate expression of the introduced sequences. This new modality of therapy might be used to replace a defective function in monogenic deficiency diseases, or to add a new function in the case of cancer and chronic viral infections. However, it is perhaps salutary to reflect that, at the time of writing, there is no clear case of a therapeutic cure or long-term remission arising out of the current gene therapy protocols. We are clearly at the stage of exploration of approaches and several features limit our ability to conduct effective therapy. Surprisingly the lack of therapeutic genes is not the immediate limiting factor; the rapid progress being made in characterizing the human genome far outstrips our ability to deliver genes to target cells and to ensure their appropriate, preferably externally, regulated expression.

Viruses, as obligatory intracellular parasites, have become the focus for exploitation as the first-generation gene therapy vectors. Four virus groups have predominated in these studies: retroviruses, herpesviruses, adenoviruses and adeno-associated viruses. Of the first 70 protocols approved by the Recombinant Advisory Committee (RAC) in the USA about 60 have involved the use of retrovirus vectors. On first examination retroviruses are not particularly promising systems as they have relatively small genomes and are limited to infecting dividing cells. However, both of these limitations are not absolute. Recently a member of a new retroviral group from fish has been sequenced and this has a proviral genome size of 12 kb (Hart and Onions, unpublished), while sequences from lentivirus *gag* proteins have been characterized that may permit the infection of resting cells. Outweighing these limitations the critical advantage that retroviruses share with adeno-associated viruses is their ability to integrate a DNA copy of their genome into chromosomal DNA so that all the progeny cells will also contain a copy of the genome.

2 The retroviral life cycle and basis of vector systems

2.1 Retroviral replication

Retroviruses belonging to the oncovirus, lentivirus and spumavirus groups have common features in their replication cycles although there are also important differences between them. All retroviruses contain two copies of a single-stranded RNA genome enclosed in a capsid, that is in turn surrounded by an envelope. Substituted into the envelope are viral glycoproteins whose external component (SU) binds to cellular receptors while viral entry is dependent on a fusion activity associated with the non-covalently linked transmembrane portion of the envelope protein. Once the virus has entered, reverse transcription of the RNA genome occurs and the resultant DNA provirus migrates to the nucleus as a nucleoprotein complex, where integration is effected by the integrase component of the reverse transcriptase complex. In gross terms, the integration of retroviruses appears random. Closer examination indicates that integration is favoured by regions of open chromatin structure characterized by high sensitivity to DNAase I. There are also indications that subsets of integration sites are non-random. Analysis of the integration sites of avian leukaemia virus (ALV) in avian cells has shown that about 20% of integrations are into one of a 1000 sites and integrations into the same site often occur at the same position (Shih *et al.*, 1988). Infection by wild-type murine (MuLV) or feline leukaemia virus (FeLV) usually leads to 1 to 30 proviral copies becoming integrated. The provirus is flanked by two long terminal repeats (LTRs) that contain the transcriptional control elements of the provirus. Between the LTRs are three main gene groups: the *gag* gene (encoding the internal structural proteins), the *pol* gene (encoding reverse transcriptase) and the *env* gene (coding for the envelope proteins). Transcription is driven from the left hand (5') LTR but it is important to note that the enhancer elements in progeny virions are derived by reiteration of the 3' LTR of the parental provirus, a feature of the replication cycle that has important consequences for vector design.

In the type C oncoviruses like MuLV and FeLV the splicing patterns are simple. A full length transcript acts as genomic RNA and as mRNA for the *gag* and *pol* genes, whereas a less abundant spliced mRNA is used to express *env*. The *env* transcripts originate at the start of R region of the LTR and in most viruses there is a splice donor site (SD) in the leader sequence upstream of *gag*. Translation of the full length transcripts results in expression of the gag, pro and pol proteins. Pro is a protease that cleaves the gag and pol poly-protein and is encoded by sequences between *gag* and *pol* although the arrangement of the reading frames encoding these sequences varies in different retrovirus subgroups. The *gag, pro* and *pol* genes form a single translational unit which is expressed as a set of nested products of the form *gag, gag-pro, gag-pro-pol*. This process ensures the production of the correct ratio of each protein, and positions the *gag* and *pol* gene products within the virion.

2.2   Basic retroviral vectors

A retroviral vector system comprises two components, a packaging line and the vector DNA construct. A packaging line is based on the observation that sequences in the leader between the 5′ LTR and the start of *gag* are necessary and sufficient for packaging oncovirus genomic RNA, although the efficiency of packaging is influenced by sequences extending beyond the packaging signal. The simplest packaging line consists of a provirus in which the packaging sequence has been deleted. When stably transfected into a cell, virus particles containing reverse transcriptase will be produced but virion RNA should not become packaged within these virions.

The complementary component of the system is a proviral form of the vector. This must of course contain a packaging sequence and certain other elements required for reverse transcription and integration of the vector (Fig. 1). However the viral structural genes may be removed and replaced with a gene of interest which can be transcribed from the LTR or from an internal promoter. Once transfected or introduced by infection into a packaging line the vector sequences will be expressed and incorporated into virions which can now infect and deliver the gene to target cells. As the vector lacks structural genes no further replication occurs (Fig. 2).

3   The safety of retroviral vectors

3.1   Replication-competent retrovirus

The simple packaging system described above is inherently unsafe. Within a very short time recombination between the vector and packaging sequence will lead to the development of replication-competent retrovirus (RCR). The contamination of vector stocks by RCR is potentially very serious and rigorous screening for these viruses under Good Laboratory Practice is essential. The recent report of Donahue *et al.* (1992) reinforces the concerns about replication-competent virus. In Donahue's study, bone marrow cells were infected with a vector preparation that contained 10^3–10^4 infectious wild-type particles ml^{-1}. The monkeys were severely immuno-compromised both by total body irradiation (500 rads × 2) and T-cell depletion from the autologous graft. Three of the eight monkeys receiving infected CD34$^+$ cells went on to develop T-cell lymphomas within 200 days.

The development of safer packaging lines has focused on reducing the recombination between the vector and the packaging construct. Second-generation packaging cell lines like pA317 improved safety by deleting the 3′ LTR in the packaging construct so that two recombination events were required to generate RCR. This cell line has been used widely in the production of gene therapy vectors but in commercial-scale production RCR has been detected in some production lots. An important step forward was made with the production of third-generation packaging lines by Danos and Mulligan (1988) and Markowitz *et al.* (1988). These lines contain the *gag-pol* genes on one construct and the *env* gene on a second so that multiple recombination events are required to generate RCR. These packaging lines are important tools in the development of gene therapy but further improvements are possible and are under investigation by our group and others. One source of concern is the overlap between the end of *pol* and the beginning of *env;* in this case recombination can be reduced by introducing codon wobbling into one of the constructs (Morgenstern

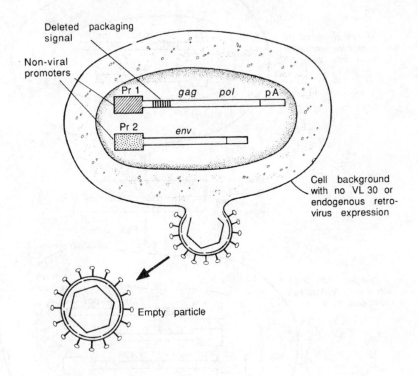

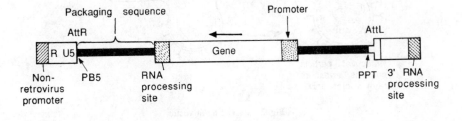

Minimal retroviral (SIN) vector

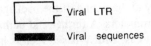

Fig. 1 Packaging line.

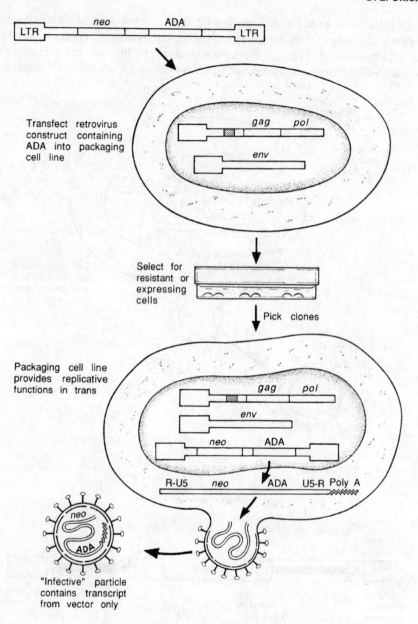

Fig. 2 Packaging of vector.

and Land, 1990). Similarly homology at the 5′ end of the packaging constructs can be reduced by using non-retroviral promoters. A further and perhaps most valuable method of reducing recombination is to use MuLV-based vectors in FeLV packaging lines and vice versa. Despite having relatively little homology between them, these viruses will package each other's genomes, presumably because of the secondary and tertiary configuration of the packaging RNA sequence (Harrison *et al.,* 1995).

3.2 Insertional mutagenesis by the vector

Integration of a vector or wild-type provirus adjacent to a cellular gene can disrupt the normal pattern of gene expression. At the simplest level, proviral integration may disrupt the gene thereby inactivating it. However, an important mode of leukaemogenesis by retroviruses involves the insertional activation of adjacent genes. This process becomes of concern when the activated gene is a proto-oncogene whose deregulation can form one of the steps towards cancer development (reviewed in Onions, 1994). Insertional activation can take several forms. In our own studies of FeLV-based leukaemogenesis the *myc* gene is a principal target. In one form of activation a defective retrovirus consisting of a 5' LTR inserts in the first intron of the gene and directs the transcription of the two coding exons. In another form the virus is upstream of the first exon and in the opposite transcriptional orientation, but transcriptional control from the *myc* promoters is under the influence of the viral enhancers in the U3 region of the LTR (Neil *et al.,* 1983; Fulton *et al.,* 1987).

Insertion of a provirus in the 3' untranslated region of a gene can also affect the stability of the mRNA. This has been observed for the *pim*-1 gene in rodent T-cell tumours induced by MuLV. In this case the insertion results in a message lacking an AUUUA motif, the net effect being to enhance the stability of the pim-1 mRNA (Shaw and Kamen, 1986). However the predominant modes of tumorogenesis clearly involve sequences in the LTR. The U3 region of the LTR contains an enhancer which may be duplicated in particular pathogenic variants of the MuLV and FeLV (Fulton *et al.,* 1990). In a typical MuLV enhancer of about 75 bp there may be binding sites for at least seven known transcription factors. The central motif within the core of the enhancer is conserved across the mammalian type C oncoviruses and consists of binding sites for LVb, core enhancer binding protein, nuclear factor 1 (Speck and Baltimore, 1987) and glucocorticoid response element (Miksicek *et al.,* 1986). The most direct method of reducing the leukaemogenicity of the vector is to remove critical elements including the enhancer from the 3' LTR in the vector introduced into the packaging cells (Fig. 1). The progeny virions will have 5' and 3' LTRs derived from this region and so will be reduced in their capacity to activate adjacent genes. Furthermore, such self-inactivating (SIN) vectors are incapable of being mobilized by superinfecting wild-type virus. However the great disadvantage of these vectors is that the titres from packaging lines are often low. Several other creative solutions to solving this problem are being investigated but one of the inherent problems is that as yet there are no simple means of testing the safety of such vectors.

The approach of infecting mice with vectors and observing the tumour incidence is not a practicable solution to safety testing; many thousands of mice would have to be infected to obtain meaningful data as multiple genetic hits are required to transform a cell. We are evaluating an alternative approach. We have produced transgenic mice with the human *myc* gene directed to express in the T-cell lineage under the control of the CD2 locus control region (LCR) or dominant control region (DCR) identified by Dimitris Kioussis and colleagues (Greaves *et al.*, 1989). Such mice develop a low incidence of T-cell neoplasia in the first year of life, as the CD2 element directs the expression of the gene in a copy-dependent and position-independent manner within the T-cell compartment. One can now determine if the vector can deliver additional oncogenic hits by infecting cells *ex vivo* and retransplanting them into syngeneic mice. Experiments with wild-type virus indicate that the superinfecting virus accelerates clonal tumour development in CD2-*myc* mice compared to that observed with the transgene or virus alone. This system, therefore, has the power to reveal low level oncogenic effects and uncover additional genes that collaborate with *myc* in leukaemogenesis (Stewart *et al.*, 1993).

3.3 Recombination of the vector with non-packaging sequences

An event unique to this class of viruses is their ability to infect the germ line stem cells and become transmitted as genetic elements called endogenous proviruses. In some strains of laboratory mice these genetically inherited viruses become expressed and eventually lead to the development of leukaemia. In most species, however, endogenous proviruses are under tight transcriptional control in the whole animal and are not usually expressed as infectious virus. A positive selection pressure for the retention of endogenous proviruses may be the property of viral interference, in which viral glycoproteins expressed within a cell block the cellular receptors and prevent superinfection.

The relationship between endogenous viruses and their horizontally transmitted exogenous counterparts can be complex. The domestic cat contains two principal sets of endogenous viruses. One group, called RD114, is closely related to an endogenous virus of baboons and is found in the germ line of all Old World cats but not in the DNA of New World cats. It has been suggested that this virus was transmitted to ancestral cat species after the division of the Old and New World species several million years ago. The second main proviral family is related to FeLV, the leukaemogenic virus of cats. Endogenous FeLV is not expressed as complete virus particles but envelope message can be detected in certain cells.

In humans there are a large number of defective proviruses divided into broad classes. Class I viruses are related to type C retroviruses like FeLV and MuLV while class II viruses have greater sequence similarity to the mammary tumour virus of mice. Until recently, it has been thought that none of these proviruses can produce infectious virus particles. However, Miller has reported a virus related to RD114 being expressed in the marrow of a patient following retroviral vector treatment (Miller, 1995). Certainly transcripts of class I proviruses have been observed in normal spleens, placentae and colon carcinomas. Similarly class I and II transcripts have been detected in breast carcinomas (Larsson *et al.*, 1989). In addition to these genetic remnants of once-infectious retroviruses, vertebrate cells contain mobile genetic elements, retroposons, that encode reverse transcriptase and can be mobile within a cell through expression of an RNA copy followed by its reverse transcription and reinsertion into another chromosomal site.

Most of the packaging lines being employed to produce vectors for gene therapy are based on murine NIH/3T3 cells and have the disadvantage that at least two classes of retroviral related sequences, VL30 and MCF, may be expressed and packaged in the vector virions. Two safety issues arise from these observations. First, can the endogenous elements be packaged into vectors and delivered to target cells? Second, can recombination occur between the vector and the endogenous sequences in the packaging line or target cell to generate novel infectious retroviruses? It is clear that VL30 sequences are packaged by vectors produced in NIH/3T3 cells and can be delivered to human cells. For this reason alone there is a need to develop safer systems with packaging lines based on well-characterized human cells. The use of human cells or other cells of non-murine origin will also contribute to overcoming the complement-dependent inactivation of oncovirus vectors which is a potential problem of their use *in vivo* (Takeuchi *et al.,* 1994). Recombination between unrelated retroviruses is known although it is rare. For instance, the Kirsten sarcoma was derived by passage of a murine leukaemia virus in rats. The resultant virus contained MuLV sequences, a transduced rat oncogene and VL30 sequences which are related to, but distinct from, infectious retrovirus genomes. These recombinations were dependent on replication-competent virus and, for a vector, one can conclude that the risk of producing novel viruses is extremely low.

4 Future developments

The future developments of retroviral vectors may be based on targeting specific functions like the specificity of infection, expression and integration and by designing systems that are crippled in their capacity to activate adjacent genes. However, technical improvements in the good manufacturing production and storage of the vector stocks will also be important in ensuring that high titred stable stocks of vectors are available for clinical use.

4.1 Targeting infection

The specificity of infection is principally governed by the envelope gene of the vector although post-entry blocks to infection are known and some have been mapped to the major capsid protein. The envelope glycoproteins may have a wider series of effects on cells than simply being passive receptors. For example, the Friend murine leukaemia virus contains a defective envelope gene product which is able to bind to and activate the erythropoietin receptor by binding to an internal site (Li *et al.,* 1990), while in contrast, FeLV-C produces one of the most acute retroviral diseases known, of a fatal pure red cell hypoplasia in which there is a rapid fall in the number of erythroid precursor cells (BFU-E) (Onions *et al.,* 1982).

Domains associated with receptor specificity have been determined from analysis of natural and laboratory-based recombinant viruses. In cats three subgroups of

FeLV, A, B and C, have been defined on the basis of their receptor usage. Subgroup A viruses are naturally transmitted from cat to cat but are unable to infect human cells. However, recombination between the subgroup A virus and endogenous FeLV sequences occurs to generate a new virus, subgroup B, which has an expanded host range and an ability to infect human cells (Stewart *et al.,* 1986). The critical changes are located to a variable region (Vr1) found at the amino terminus of the surface unit (SU) of the envelope protein. Similarly, mutations within this variable domain are responsible for changing a subgroup A virus to one with subgroup C specificity which is able to infect human cells through a different receptor from FeLV-B (Rigby *et al.,* 1992). Similar domains are found within the murine retroviruses and these amino terminal regions of FeLV and MuLV provide potential sites for engineering receptor specificity (Battini *et al.,* 1995).

The receptor for FeLV-B on human cells has been shown to be identical to that for gibbon ape leukaemia virus (GaLV), although these viruses have little homology in their receptor binding domain regions (Takeuchi *et al.,* 1992). The GaLV/FeLV-B receptor (GLVR1) is a sodium-dependent phosphate symporter. Surprisingly, amphotropic MuLV (A-MuLV), which forms the basis of the widely used packaging lines, also uses a related but distinct phosphate symporter (Ram1) (Kavanaugh *et al.,* 1994). There are suggestions that the density of the GLVR1 receptor is higher on CD34$^+$ cells than Ram1 so that vectors with the GaLV/FeLV-B receptor specificity may have a particular role in transduction into haemopoietic stem cells. Moreover as these are induceable receptors, manipulation of the culture conditions of haemopoietic cells may enable increased transduction efficiencies to be obtained.

Receptor specificity may also be altered by incorporating envelope genes of other viruses into the packaging line based on MuLV or FeLV. The most promising system is that developed by Friedmann and his colleagues based on vesicular stomatitis virus (Emi *et al.,* 1991; Friedmann and Yee, 1995). The VSV-G gene encodes a glycoprotein that interacts with phosphatidyl serine and possibly other components of the bilayer present on most cells, so that vectors with this envelope glycoprotein can efficiently enter all vertebrate cells and even invertebrate cells. However, the outstanding advantage of these vectors is that they are very robust and can be concentrated to much higher titres (10^8–10^9 infectious units ml^{-1}) than can be achieved with conventional vectors.

More radical methods of altering receptor specificity have been approached through the addition of specific ligand coding regions into the amino-terminal variable region of the SU protein. Packaging systems containing chimeric envelope genes encoding single chain antigen binding site of an antibody have been shown to produce virions that will bind specifically to the target antigen although they were unable to infect cells expressing these antigens (Russel *et al.,* 1993). Recently, infectious viruses with altered receptor specificity have been produced. In Kasahara's study the entire sequence encoding human erythropoietin was substituted into the amino-terminus of an MuLV *env* gene and the virions containing this modified envelope gene were able to infect HeLa cells expressing a transfected *Epo* receptor but not the control cells (Kasahara *et al.,* 1994). Similarly, a single chain antibody fragment specific for an antigen on human colon carcinoma cells was shown to confer appropriate specificity on vector virions (Chu and Dornberg, 1995). In both cases effective delivery required the co-presence of the ecotropic MuLV envelope glyco-protein, presumably to provide appropriate fusion of the viral envelope with the cel-lular membrane. These results are promising but some caution is required, since the titres of these modified viruses is extremely low and far removed from that required for therapeutic purposes.

4.2 Targeting expression

A major limiting factor of retroviral vectors as agents for introducing genes into pluripotential stem cells is down-regulation of expression. The mechanisms for this are uncertain but are influenced by regulatory elements within the LTR and by sequences around the primer binding site in the untranslated leader sequence. Position effects of integration and the properties of specific genes within the vector also influence suppression. A concomitant of these processes is methylation of the LTR which probably determines the long-term suppression of transcription.

Expressing two genes like a selectable marker and a therapeutic gene can result in cross-interference in some vectors; so the trend is towards single gene vector sys-tems. Future developments may include the incorporation of locus-defining sequences (Grosveld et al., 1987) that can target expression to particular tissue com-partments like the CD2 control region, used to target transgene expression to T-cells (Greaves et al., 1989; Stewart et al., 1993). However, a limiting factor of most cur-rently defined LCRs is the extensive size of these elements required to ensure posi-tion-independent and copy number-dependent expression. Recent data suggest that for at least some LCRs the enhancer domain must be bilaterally flanked by extensive (1 kb) domains termed 'facilitators' (Aronow et al., 1995).

4.3 Targeting integration

Many of the limiting features of retrovirus vectors could be overcome if directed tar-geting of the vector could be achieved. Some retroviral related elements like the yeast retrotransposon Ty3 display remarkable fidelity of integration. In the case of Ty3, integration occurs precisely into the five base pairs at the start of transcription of Pol III transcribed genes. Recently, Kirchner et al. (1995) have shown that the transcription factors TFIIIB and TFIIIC are necessary to enable position-specific integration. Similar studies in HIV have indicated that integration may be dependent on interaction between the viral integrase complex and a DNA binding protein des-ignated ini I (Kalpana et al., 1995). The tethering of the integrase to specific tran-scription factors may open up a route to the targeting of integration. In an exciting demonstration of this concept, Bushman (1994) has demonstrated targeted integra-tion in an in vitro system. The HIV integrase was modified by fusion to a λ phage repressor DNA binding domain and it was found that integration directed by the hybrid molecule was biased towards repressor binding sites.

5 Conclusion

When gene therapy finally comes of age it is unlikely that any of the vectors in their current form will be in use. Future vector systems may be synthetic and capable of manufacture on a large scale but will incorporate viral-like elements to ensure their effective delivery. One can envision large plasmid vectors regulated by LCRs and maintained in episomal form or integrated using viral enzyme machinery. To ensure their entry into cells they would possess ligand binding receptors together with viral fusion elements to permit effective exit of the construct from the endosome. However, in the medium term, viral vectors have much to offer and retrovirus vectors will predominate in systems aimed at introducing genes into haemopoietic stem cells.

References

Aronow, B. J., Ebert, C. A., Valerius, M. T., Potter, S. S., Wiginton, D. A., Witte, D. P. and Hutton, J. J. (1995). *Mol. Cell. Biol.* **15**, 1123–1135.

Battini, J.-L., Danos, O. and Heard, J. M. (1995). *J. Virol.* **69**, 713–719.

Bushman, F. D. (1994). *Proc. Natl. Acad. Sci. USA.* **91**, 9233–9237.

Chu, T.-H.T. and Dornburg, R. (1995). *J. Virol.* **69**, 2659-2663.

Danos, O. and Mulligan, R. C. (1988). *Proc. Natl. Acad. Sci. USA* **85**, 6460–6464.

Donahue, R. E., Kessler, S. W., Bodine, D., McDonagh, K., Dunbar, C., Goodman, S., Agricola, B., Byrne, E., Raffeld, M., Moen, R., Bacher, J., Zsebo, K. M. and Nienhuis, A. W. (1992). *J. Exp. Med.* **176**, 1125–1135.

Emi, N., Friedmann, T. and Yee, J.-K. (1991). *J. Virol.* **65**, 1212–1207.

Friedmann, T. and Yee, J.-K. (1995). *Nature Med.* **1**, 275–277.

Fulton, R., Forrest, D., Mcfarlane, R., Onions, D. and Neil, J. C. (1987). *Nature* **326**, 190–194.

Fulton, R., Plumb, M., Shield, L. and Neil, J.C. (1990). *J. Virol.* **64**, 1675–1682.

Greaves, D. R., Wilson, F. D., Lang, G. and Kioussis, D. (1989). *Cell* **56**, 979–986.

Grosveld, F., van Assendelft, G., Greaves, D. R. and Kollias, G. (1987). *Cell* **51**, 975–985.

Harrison, G. P., Hunter, E. and Lever, A. M. L. (1995). *J. Virol.* **69**, 2175–2186.

Kalpana, G. V., Marmon, S., Wang, W., Crabtree, G. R. and Goff, S.P. (1995). *Science* **266**, 2002–2006.

Kasahara, N., Dozy, A. M. and Kan, Y. W. (1994). *Science* **266**, 1373–1375.

Kavanaugh, M. P., Miller, D. G., Zhang, W., Law, W., Kozak, S. L., Kabat, D. and Miller, A. D. (1994). *Proc. Natl. Acad. Sci. USA* **91**, 7071–7075.

Kirchner, J., Connolly, C. M. and Sandmeyer, S. B. (1995). *Science* **267**, 1488–1491.

Larson, E., Kato, N. and Cohen, M. (1989). *Curr. Topics Microbiol. Immunol.* **148**, 115–132.

Li, J. P., D'andrea, A. D., Lodish, H. F. and Baltimore, D. (1990). *Nature* **343**, 762–764.

Markowitz, D., Goff, S. and Bank, A. (1988) *Virology* **167**, 400–406.

Miksicek, R., Heber, A., Schmid, W., Danesch, U., Posseckert, G., Beato, M. and Schutz, G. (1986). *Cell* **46**, 283–290.

Miller (1995). *Science* (in press).

Morgenstern, J. P. and Land, H. (1990). *Nucl. Acids Res.* **18**, 3587–3596.

Neil, J. C., Hughes, R., McFarlane, R., Onions, D. E., Lees, G. and Jarrett, O. (1983). *Nature* **208**, 814–20.

Onions, D., Jarrett, O., Testa, N., Frassoni, F. and Toth, S. *Nature* **296**, 156–8.

Onions, D. E. (1994). In *Haematological Oncology Cambridge Medical Reviews*, Vol 3. (A. Burnett, J. Armitage, A. Newland and A. Keating eds), pp. 35–72. Cambridge University Press, Cambridge.

Rigby, M. A., Rojko, J. L., Stewart, M. A., Kociba, G. J., Cheney, C. M., Rezanka, L. J., Mathes, L. E., Hartke, J. R., Jarrett, O. and Neil, J. C. (1992). *J. Gen. Virol.* **73**, 2839–2847.

Russell, S. J., Hawkins, R. E. and Winter, G. (1993). *Nucl. Acids Res.* **21**, 1081–1108.

Shaw, G. and Kamen, R. (1986). *Cell* **46**, 659–667.

Speck, N. A. and Baltimore, D. (1987). *Mol. Cell Biol.* **7**, 1101–1110.

Stewart, M. A., Warnock, M., Wheeler, A., Wilkie, N., Mullins, J. I., Onions, D. E. and Neil, J. C. (1986). *J. Virol.* **58**, 825–834.

Stewart, M., Cameron, E., Campbell, M., McFarlane, R., Toth, S., Lang, K., Onions, D. and Neil, J. C. (1993). *Int. J. Cancer* **53**, 1023–1030.

Takeuchi, Y., Vile, R. G., Simpson, G., O'Hara, B., Collins, M. K. and Weiss, R. A. (1992). *J. Virol.* **66**, 1219–1222.

Takeuchi, Y., Cosset, F.-L., Lachmann, P. J., Okada, H., Weiss, R. A. and Collins, M. (1994). *J. Virol.* **68**, 8001–8007.

Appendix: Abstracts of Posters

Contents

Genome Projects

Interpreting the Code

From Gene to Target

From Target to Therapy

Genome Projects

Mapping the Swine Genome: Current Status and Future Directions.

L. B. Schook[1], A. A. Paszek[1], C. F. Louis[1], C. W. Beattie[2], G. A. Rohrer[2], L. J. Alexander[2] and M. B. Wheeler[3]. *Department of Veterinary Pathobiology, University of Minnesota, St Paul, MN;* [2]*Gene Mapping/Expression Group, RL Hruska US Meat Animal Research Center (MARC), Clay Center, NE;* [3]*Department of Animal Sciences, University of Illinois, Urbana, IL, USA*

A collaborative mapping effort between the USDA, ARS, Roman L. Hruska US Meat Animal Research Center (MARC) and the University of Minnesota was established to integrate physical and genetic linkage maps of the pig and map loci associated with disease resistance, growth and development, and carcass traits. These efforts are supported by construction of a microsatellite linkage map of the pig [1] using exotic Chinese germplasm crossed to conventional US breeding stock (MARC and the University of Illinios). It is expected that the maps will aid in the identification of genetic markers which can be incorporated into a marker-assisted selection breeding programme [2,3]. Allelic frequencies for framework microsatellites in commercial breeds have also been determined. The first swine chromosome workshop [4] devoted to a single chromosome developed a framework and comprehensive map of chromosome 6, and led to the organization of a workshop focused on swine chromosome 7, set for later this year. Physical mapping efforts are centred on assigning cosmid and lambda genomic clones containing informative microsatellites using fluorescent *in situ* hybridization (FISH). We are selecting a set of framework markers (based on heterozygosity, quality of amplified product and physical location) which can be incorporated into automated flourescent genotyping protocols useful for QTL mapping in most swine resource populations.

[1] Rohrer, G. A. *et al.* (1994). *Genetics* **136** 231–245.
[2] Schook, L. B. *et al.* (1994). *Anim. Biotechnol.* **5** 129–135.
[3] Schook, L. B. *et al.* (1995). *J. Anim. Sci.* (in press).
[4] Paszek, A. A. *et al.* (1995). *Anim. Genet.* (in press).

Evidence for a Susceptibility Locus for Schizophrenia on Chromosome 22q.

David Collier, Homero Vallada, Michael Gill and the Schizophrenia Collaborative Linkage Group (Chromosome 22). *Institute of Psychiatry, DeCrespigny Park, Denmark Hill, London SE5 8AF, UK*

Several groups have reported weak evidence for linkage between schizophrenia and genetic markers located on chromosome 22q using the lod score method of analysis. However these findings involved different genetic markers and methods of analysis, and so were not directly comparable. To resolve this issue we have performed a combined analysis of genotypic data from the marker D22S278 in multiply affected schizophrenic families derived from 11 independent research groups worldwide. This marker was chosen because it showed maximum evidence for linkage in two independent datasets and maps to 22q12 between D22S268 and IL2RB, two markers previously reported as potentially linked to schizophrenia but not confirmed by a combined lod score analysis. Using the affected sib pair method as implemented by the program ESPA, the combined dataset showed 252 alleles shared compared with 188 alleles not shared (chi-square 9.31, 1 df, $P = 0.001$) where parental genotype data was completely known. When sib pairs for whom parental data was assigned according to probability were included the number of alleles shared was 514.1 compared with 437.8 not shared (chi-square 6.12, 1 df, $P = 0.006$). Similar results were obtained when a likelihood ratio method for sib pair analysis was used. These results provide evidence of a susceptibility locus of moderate effect on liability to develop schizophrenia at 22q12.

Molecular Cloning of a DNAase-1–like Gene Located on the Human X Chromosome. Valentina Appierto, Rossana Pergolizzi, Alessandro Bosetti, Laura Bianchi, GianLuca DeBellis, Ermanna Rovida and Ida Biunno. *Istituto Tecnologie Biomediche Avanzate, CNR Via Ampère 56, 20131 Milano, Italy*

The human genome project will provide the sequence of many genes of unknown function. Identification of new genes is a very difficult task and requires the simultaneous application of several methods. Using the direct cDNA selection approach, we have recently isolated a full length cDNA named Xib whose sequence analysis showed good homology to the DNAase-1 gene family. Xib maps on the q28 region of the human X chromosome, in the G6PD locus. ZOO blot analysis showed a remarkable cross-species conservation of Xib, in fact DNA fragments were seen in organisms as far distant as fish. Northern blot analysis indicated the preferential expression of this gene in the cardioskeletal system; alternative splicing was also observed in some fetal tissues. By virtue of Xib chromosomal localization and specific expression we sought to find a relationship with two muscle-associated disorders described in this region: Emery–Dreifuss and Barth syndromes. No gross chromosomal deletions were observed in patients' DNA. Data will be presented on the homology between Xib and the DNAase-1 enzyme.

Automated Sequencing of Viral Genome in Blood Samples for Clinical Diagnosis. Chwan-Heng Wang[1] and Shu-Yuan Tschen[2]. *[1]Abteilung für Medizinische Virologie und Epidemiologie der Viruskrankheiten, Hygiene Institut der Eberhard-Karls Universität Tübingen, Silcherstr. 7, D-72076 Tübingen; [2]Institut für Mikrobiologie I der Eberhard-Karls Universität Tübingen, Auf der Morgenstelle 28, D-72076 Tübingen, Germany*

The use of polymerase chain reaction (PCR) and DNA sequencing has recently become a powerful tool for diagnosis of blood-borne infectious agents and has potential clinical application. For example, identification (subtyping) of hepatitis B virus (HBV) genomes circulating in blood was thought to be essential in assessment of infectivity, chronicity and monitoring efficiency of interferon therapy. Recently, we have developed a simple, rapid and quantitative amplification of the HBV genomes in serum samples. Using this principle, detection (by PCR) and subtyping (by DNA sequencing or hybridization) of viral antigen with different primers specifically pairing to different viral genome regions can be combined for automation. In this report, we describe our development in this automated sequencing procedure designed for the molecular diagnosis by subtyping and sequencing of whole viral genome directly from blood sample. Further generalization of this automatic detection to other blood-borne viruses for clinical use will be discussed.

Interpreting the Code

Cloning and Expression of a Novel Lipoprotein-associated Phospholipase A₂ (Lp-PLA₂).

G. Mark, P. Lawrence[1], Simon Q. J. Rice[1], Colin H. MacPhee[2], Christopher D. Southan[2], Haodong Li[3], David G. Tew[2], Helen Saul[2], Kitty Moores[3] and Isro S. Gloger[1]. *[1]SmithKline Beecham Pharmaceuticals, New Frontiers Science Park, Third Avenue, Harlow CM19 5AW, UK; [2]SmithKline Beecham Pharmaceuticals, The Frythe, Welwyn, Herts AL6 9AR, UK; [3]Human Genome Science, Rockville, MD, USA*

We have cloned and expressed the cDNA for a novel phospholipase A₂(Lp-PLA₂) by homology screening of a λ ZAP cDNA library. Using peptide sequences derived from proteolytic fragments of Lp-PLA₂ that has been purified from human plasma, three previously 'unknown' ESTs from the HGS database were identified that could potentially code for these sequences. One of these EST clones was radiolabelled and used to reprobe the library to isolate the full-length Lp-PLA₂ cDNA. The DNA sequence was determined for the full-length clone. The predicted size for protein expressed from the putative open reading frame was in good agreement with experimental results on purified enzyme. The proteolytic fragment sequences could be found in the translated sequence. The full-length cDNA was inserted into a suitable expression vector and expressed in both transient and stable mammalian systems. The expressed Lp-PLA₂ showed activity in a ³[H]PAF assay and the enzyme was inhibited by known inhibitors. In addition the recombinant Lp-PLA₂ was successfully immunoprecipitated with a polyclonal antibody raised against the native enzyme.

An Automated Method for Calculating Scoring Matrices and Gap Penalties for Sequence Alignment.

Mor Amitai. *Institute of Mathematics and Centre for Rationality and Interactive Decision Theory, The Hebrew University, Jerusalem and Compugen Ltd, 17 Hamacabim St, Petach-Tikva, 49220 Israel*

We describe here an approach for calculating scoring matrices and gap penalties, assuming no knowledge of relations between amino acid sequences in a given database (families) and no evolutionary model. This approach can easily be used for new databases and for building special scoring matrices and gap penalties for certain families. We use the Smith–Waterman local alignment algorithm, with the identity scoring matrix, to calculate the alignment between many sequences in the database. From these alignments, we calculate the empirical distribution of aligned pairs of amino acids and the empirical distribution of gaps. Based on these distributions we derive a scoring matrix, a gap-open penalty and a gap-extended penalty. We tested the resulting matrix and gap penalties by running 36 sequences from 12 different families against Swiss-Prot. The results show that the gap penalties, calculated from the empirical distribution of gaps, are the best gap penalties for the new matrix, and that the performance of the new matrix is equivalent to the performance of Blosum62 and better than the performance of Pam250.

Sensitive and Comprehensive Sequence Database Searching.
Oliver Bayliss[1] and Neil Rowlands[2]. *[1]Oxford Molecular Group plc, The Magdalen Centre, Oxford Science Park, Sandford-on-Thames, Oxford OX4 4GA, UK. [2]MasPar Computer Limited, 8 Commerce Park, Brunel Road, Theale, Reading, Berks RG7 4AB, UK*

The major public sequence data banks—Genbank, EMBL, DDBJ and Swiss-Prot—are growing rapidly from the efforts of the genome sequencing projects. Accompanying the growth of both public and proprietary data banks is the need for more sophisticated and sensitive tools to search them. As the volume of data increases, so does the number and similarity of random matches to a query. Rigorous searching methods are required to distinguish significant matches from background noise, and these methods must be applied to the most comprehensive set of sequence data available. Some of the popular searching tools are compared showing how an optimized implementation of the Smith–Waterman algorithm yields the most thorough examination of sequence data, improving the identification of familial and structural relationships.

Coding Sequence Dependence on the Ability of d^2 to make Novel DNA Sequence Functional Assignment.
Winston Hide, John Burke and Daniel Davison. *MasPar Computer Corporation and University of Houston, Houston, TX, USA*

A number of algorithms exist for searching sequence databases for biologically significant similarities based on primary sequence similarity of aligned sequences. We present here a high performance comparison algorithm, d^2, that rapidly determines the relative dissimilarity of large datasets of DNA sequences. We outline the ability of d^2 to detect functional motifs within DNA sequences that are indicative of gene function, and analyse the relationship of functional similarity detection with respect to the placement of the words inside and outside of coding regions. We have determined that d^2 is uniquely capable of detecting significant functional similarities between sequences that have no measurable alignable sequence similarity. Querying with a lipoprotein lipase DNA sequence results in hits that share functional similarity, such as DNA sequences coding for proteins that regulate lipid metabolism, membrane and fat interaction and lipogenesis. d^2 uses sequence–word multiplicity as a simple measure of dissimilarity. It is not constrained by the comparison of direct sequence alignments and so can use word contexts to yield new functional information on relationships. d^2 is unique in that subsequences of biological interest can be weighted to improve sensitivity and selectivity of a search over existing methods. We have determined the ability of d^2 to detect biologically significant matches between a query and large datasets of DNA sequences while varying parameters such as word length and window size. We have optimized parameters to present maximal sensitivity and selectivity relative to FASTA.

From Gene to Target

Use of Differential Display RT-PCR to study the Mechanism of Enhancement of Pre-adipocyte Differentiation by BRL 49653.

J. C. Clapham[1], M. T. McHale[2], G. C. Sibbring[1], J. C. Holder[1], S. A. Smith[1] and I. S. Gloger[2]. *[1]Department of Vascular Biology, SmithKline Beecham Pharmaceuticals, The Frythe, Welwyn, Herts AL6 9AR, UK; [2]BioPharm R&D, SmithKline Beecham Pharmaceuticals, NFSP-N, Harlow, Essex CM19 5AD, UK*

BRL 49653 [(±)-5-[(4-[2-methyl-2-(pyridinylamino)ethoxy]phenyl)methyl]2,4-thiazolidine-dione-(z)-2-butenedioate(1:1)] is a potent and selective oral antidiabetic agent [1]. It enhances tissue sensitivity to insulin and thus offers potential for the treatment of non-insulin-dependent diabetes mellitus (NIDDM). Thiazolidine-2,4-diones, as a class, also enhance insulin- or IGF-1-induced differentiation of pre-adipocytes to adipocytes *in vitro* [2]. In this study, we used the technique of reverse transcriptase differential display PCR (DD RT-PCR) [3] to identify possible early changes in gene expression in NIH 3T3-L1 fibroblasts treated with BRL −49653 under normal culture conditions (DMEM and 10% FCS). Cells were incubated with BRL 49653 (10 µmol l⁻¹) for 0, 10, 20, 30 and 120 min. Total RNA was extracted and subjected to DD RT-PCR. All PCR reactions were performed in duplicate and repeated on separate gels in order to verify potential differences. Nineteen 5′ random primers yielded a total of only 10 reproducible band differences. Several bands appeared to be induced after only 10 min of exposure to BRL 49653. Differentially displaying bands were excised and reamplified. Northern blot and DNA sequence analysis are under way. Identification of the novel products should help in elucidating the mechanism of action of BRL 49653.

[1] Cantello, B. C. C. *et al.* (1994). *J. Med. Chem.* **37**, 3977–3985.
[2] Kletzien, R. F., Clarke, S. T. and Ulrich, R. G. (1992). *Mol. Pharmacol.* **41**, 393–398.
[3] Liang, P. and Pardee, A. B. (1992). *Science*, **257**, 967–971.

Analysis of Gene Expression in Rat Brain by Differential Display Following Chronic Administration of Antidepressant Drugs.

A. Volenec, T. P. Flanigan, N. R. Newberry, J. M. Elliott, J. M. Moorman and R. A. Leslie. *Oxford University SmithKline Beecham Centre for Applied Neuropsychobiology, University Department of Clinical Pharmacology, Radcliffe Infirmary, Woodstock Road, Oxford OX2 6HE, UK*

The mechanism(s) of action underlying clinical efficacy of antidepressant drugs, such as the selective serotonin reuptake inhibitors (SSRIs), are presumed to involve neuroadaptive responses that probably include alterations in gene expression. It has been difficult to identify candidate genes that may be involved in this neuroadaptation. The technique of differential display of mRNA has been used successfully to detect and characterize known, as well as novel genes that are differentially expressed in a variety of normal physiological and pathological processes [1,2]. We are currently using differential display to investigate gene expression in the brain following chronic treatment of adult rats with antidepressant drugs.

Animals were injected subcutaneously with paroxetine (5 mg kg^{-1}, $n = 5$), fluoxetine (10 mg kg^{-1}, $n = 5$) or vehicle (5% (w/v) sucrose, $n = 5$) once daily for 21 days. Brains were removed, cerebella discarded and total RNA prepared. Reverse transcriptase-linked polymerase chain reactions were then performed in the presence of radiolabelled nucleotide and various primer combinations. DNA products were visualized on autoradiographs following separation on conventional sequencing gels and band patterns compared. Relative to vehicle, the majority of bands were unaltered following treatment with SSRIs. A number of candidate bands were detected that appeared to be up- or down-regulated by one or both SSRIs. We are currently investigating the nature of these differentially expressed bands.

This study indicates that differential display can be used to identify candidate bands, whose expression appears to be altered following chronic administration of antidepressants. This should facilitate the identification of genes that may be involved in the mechanism of action of these drugs and help explain their clinical efficacy.

[1] Liang, P. and Pardee, A. B. (1992). *Science* 257, 967–971.
[2] Sager, R., Anisowicz, A., Neveu, M., Liang, P. and Sotiropoulou, G. (1993). *FASEB J.* 7, 964–970.

Carbamazepine is a Blocker of a Rat Brain Calcium Channel Complex Expressed in *Xenopus* Oocytes.

W. J. Tomlinson. *Department of Biotechnology, University of British Columbia, British Columbia, Canada*

Carbamazepine has been widely used in the management of affective psychoses [1,2] and in the treatment of certain types of epilepsies [3]. Electrophysiological studies have shown that clinically relevant concentrations of carbamazepine can reduce the calcium-dependent component of action potentials in sensory spinal ganglion cells [4]. Carbamazepine has also been shown to have synergistic effects with verapamil (an L-type calcium channel antagonist) in decreasing calcium currents in guinea-pig hippocampal slices [5].

In neurons, rapid entry of calcium mediates many cellular responses including neurotransmitter release, hormonal secretion and gene expression [6]. The major conduit for the rapid entry of calcium into these cells is through voltage-gated calcium channels. Voltage-gated calcium channels are large transmembrane protein complexes consisting of five subunits (α_1, α_2, β, δ and γ). The α_1 subunit, of which there are several isoforms, contains both the voltage sensor and ion-conducting pore while the ancillary subunits perform a modulatory role.

α_{1C-II} is a cloned rat brain calcium channel that represents the major L-type α_1 subunit found in the rat brain [7]. In this study we examined functional interaction between carbamazepine and α_{1C-II} or α_{1C-II} + β_{1b} in a *Xenopus* oocyte expression system. Using two-electrode voltage clamps we found that carbamazepine (10 μM) is a potent inhibitor of calcium currents in *Xenopus* oocytes expressing α_{1C-II} + β_{1b}. However, when α_{1C-II} was expressed alone carbamazepine (up to 100 μM) had little or no effect on the introduced calcium currents.

The calcium channel α_1 subunit is the major target of all therapeutic agents acting at L-type calcium channels examined to date even though calcium channels are multisubunit complexes *in vivo*. Since identical α_1 subunits are found in many different tissues, this targeting of the α_1 subunit may account for many of the adverse side effects associated with traditional calcium channel inhibitory drugs. In contrast, carbamazepine appears to modulate calcium channel complexes rather than the α_1 subunit specifically. This is the first example of such pharmacological modulation of calcium channel complexes and may represent a more selective approach than α_1 subunit-directed ligands.

[1] Elphick, M. (1989). *Psychol. Med.* **19**, 591–604.
[2] Post, R. M. (1990). In *Reviews of Psychiatry*, 9th edn (A. Tasman, S. M. Goldfinger and C. A. Kaufman, eds), pp. 170–202. American Psychiatric Press, Washington, DC.
[3] *Goodman and Gilman's The Pharmacological Basis of Therapeutics*, 7th edn (1985). Macmillan, New York.
[4] Schirrmacher, K., Mayer, A., Walden, J., Dusing, R. and Bingmann, D. (1993). *Neuropsychobiology* **27**, 176–179.
[5] Walden, J., Grunze, H., Bingmann, D., Liu Z. and Dusing, R. (1992). *Eur. Neuropsychopharmacol.* **2**, 455–462.
[6] Miller, R. J. (1987). *Science* **235**, 46–52.
[7] Snutch, T. P., Tomlinson, W. J., Leonard, J. P. and Gilbert, M. M. (1991). *Neuron.* **7**, 45–57.

Cloning and Expression of the Human 5-HT$_{2b}$ Receptor, Using Extracellular Acidification Rates as a Rapid, Sensitive Measure of Receptor Functionality: a Paradigm for 'Orphan' Receptors. J. K. Chambers, J. Carey, O. Murphy, D. Gale, A. Muir, G. Baxter, M. J. Browne and S. Wilson. *SmithKline Beecham Pharmaceuticals, New Frontiers Science Park, Third Avenue, Harlow, Essex CM19 5AW, UK*

A partial cDNA clone was isolated from a human small intestine cDNA library using a probing strategy based on the rat cDNA sequence and the predicted genomic structure of the mouse homologue. The remainder of the gene was isolated from a human genomic library. The ORF of 1443 bp encodes a protein of 481 amino acids and is identical to that described recently [1]. It was subcloned into a mammalian expression vector under the control of the CMV promoter, and stable HEK293 cell transfectants selected using G418.

As the receptor was novel, it was not clear what second messenger system(s) the receptor might activate, nor what assay methodology was appropriate to assess functionality. We therefore evaluated a 'generic approach' to this problem, based on agonist stimulation of cells and the measurement of changes in extracellular acidification rates.

Mass cultures of HEK293 cells responded to 100 nM 5-HT with increased extracellular acidification rates as measured using the Cytosensor™ microphysiometer. Control cells did not respond. One mass culture was selected for cloning on the basis that it produced the largest increase in acidification rates. A single dilution clone was selected for further study on the same basis. Testing of each culture required only 0.3 million cells.

Quantitative, reproducible, dose-dependent responses to 5-HT (pEC_{50} = 7.5 (7.3–8.0), n = 10) were maximal within 2 min and no desensitization was apparent upon repeated administration of a single concentration of agonist. The 5-HT$_{2b}$ antagonist SB204741 gave an apparent pA_2 value of 7.49 (7.26–7.82), n = 4: similar to affinity estimates at the rat 5-HT$_{2b}$ receptor (pA_2 = 7.95) [2].

This strategy thus provides a rapid and sensitive means to select stable cell lines and evaluate the functionality of novel receptors in the absence of detailed foreknowledge of coupling specificity.

[1] Schmuck, K. *et al.* (1994). *FEBS Lett.* **342**, 85–90.
[2] Baxter, G. *et al.* (1995). *Br. J. Pharmacol.* (in press).

From Target to Therapy

Inhibitors and Mechanism of Bacterial Translocase I, a Cell Wall Biosynthetic Enzyme. P. E. Brandish[1], T. D. H. Bugg[1], J. Lonsdale[2], M. Black[2] and R. Southgate[2]. *Department of Chemistry, University of Southampton, Southampton, Hants, UK; 2SmithKline Beecham Pharmaceuticals, Brockham Park, Betchworth, Surrey RH3 7AJ, UK*

Bacterial cell wall biosynthesis represents a good target for novel compounds in the on-going search for effective therapeutic antibiotics. The current project is a study of the title enzyme which catalyses the first step in the membrane cycle of reactions in peptidoglycan biosynthesis. The mode of action of the specific inhibitors mureidomycin A and liposidomycin B is under investigation.

The *Escherichia coli mraY* gene has been overexpressed in the strain *E. coli* JM109 (pBROC525), giving 80-fold enzyme overexpression. Enzyme activity has been solubilized from membrane fragments using the detergent Triton X-100. A continuous fluorescence enhancement assay has been developed using a substrate carrying a fluorophore in the peptide chain permitting detailed kinetic studies. Preliminary results suggest that mureidomycin A functions as a slow-binding reversible inhibitor with K_i = 39 nM, as characterized by a biphasic time course in the presence of inhibitor.

Amino acid sequence alignments suggest that translocase I is a member of a family of membrane-linked phospho-sugar transferases which includes eukaryotic enzymes involved in dolichol phosphate-linked glycoprotein biosynthesis. Based on sequence alignments and biochemical data we propose that Asp 267 may function as a catalytic residue, and that Asp 115 and Asp 116 may be part of a Mg^{2+}-pyrophosphate binding domain. These roles are under investigation using site-directed mutagenesis.

Solubilization of overexpressed enzyme, development of a convenient assay system and site-directed mutagenesis have provided the tools for an in-depth mechanistic analysis of this enzyme.

CD34+ Cells from Thawed Peripheral Blood are Increased by Phosphorothioate Antisense TGF-β1 in Liquid Culture.

A. Grosse[1], O. Feugeas[1,2], C. Coutton[1], P. Furstenberger[1,2,3], I. Rusciani[1,2,3] and F. Oberling[1,2]. [1]*Institut d'Hématologie et* [3]*Eurothera, Hospices Civils, 1 Place de l'Hôpital,* [2]*Service d'Onco-Hématologie, Hôpital de Hautepierre, 67000 Strasbourg, France*

Advantages of peripheral blood stem cells (PBSC) over the use of autologous bone marrow include a reduced risk of tumour cell contamination, the ability to collect PBSC without general anaesthesia, and a rapid haematopoietic recovery. But, in spite of using growth factors, the proportion of PBSC still remains low because of myeloablative therapy, and two to five leukaphereses during several days are necessary to collect sufficient PBSC for a rapid and sustained haematopoietic recovery after transplantation.

Antisense TGF-β1 phosphorothioate oligodeoxynucleotides increased more than cytokines alone the number of CD34+ isolated from fresh normal bone marrow and umbilical cord blood [1]. We have tested the proliferative effect of antisense TGF-β1 on haematopoietic CD34+ stem cells isolated from thawed, mobilized and aphereses-collected PBSC of patients with a variety of malignancies (lymphoma and myeloma) or from normal bone marrow.

Low density mononuclear stem cells were processed using the Ceprate LC CD34 Kit (CellPro). Purified CD34+ cells were cultured in liquid medium for 72 h in the presence of cytokines (IL-3, IL-6, G-CSF, GM-CSF, SCF) and with antisense, sense or missense TGF-β1. The effect of antisense was tested by CD34 and CD38 labelling, by clonogenic assays (CFU-GM and BFU-E), and by study of cell cycle using DNA flow cytometric analysis. Only less than 10% of purified CD34+ cells were CD38-.

This study showed a great maturation of the progenitor CD34+ cells when cultured *in vitro* in the presence of our cytokine combination: only 58.2% of the 90.5% CD34+ cells collected after being immunopurified were still CD34+. The addition of antisense TGF-β1 to the culture medium seemed to speed up this maturation: only 40.8% of cells remained CD34+ after 72 h. Effects in the same direction were observed when the CD38 stainings were analysed.

Compared with the growth factors alone, addition of antisense TGF-β1 increases 1.8- and 2.15-fold the number of CFU-GM and BFU-E, respectively. No effects were observed when sense or missense was added to the medium.

Our results show that antisense TGF-β1 increases CD34+ cells, in the case of CD34+ isolated from either the bone marrow or the PBSC. These results obtained from PBSC suggest a future potential use of these *in vitro* expansion techniques as part of neoplastic treatments.

[1] Hatzfeld, J. *et al.* (1991). *J. Exp. Med.* **174**, 925–929.

Identification of a Phenylethanolamine with High Efficacy at Human Cloned β_3-Adrenoceptors (β_3-AR) that Stimulates Human White Adipocyte Lipolysis via β_3-AR.

M. V. Sennitt[2], L. J. Beeley[1], J. M. Berge[1], H. Chapman[1], M. A. Cawthorne[1], J. Kelly[1], S. A. Smith[1], M. J. Stock[2], S. Wilson[1], P. W. Young[1] and J. R. S. Arch[1]. [1]*SmithKline Beecham Pharmaceuticals, The Frythe, Welwyn, Herts AL6 9AR, UK;* [2]*St George's Hospital Medical School, Tooting, London SW17 0RE, UK*

Although β_3-AR mRNA has been detected in human adipose and gastrointestinal tissues, there is limited evidence that β_3-AR can mediate functional responses in human tissues. Moreover, this evidence is primarily that the aryloxypropanolamine CGP 12177 elicits responses that are poorly blocked by standard β-AR antagonists: lipolytic responses to phenylethanolamine agonists, such as isoprenaline or BRL 37344, are well blocked and appear to be mediated by β_1 or β_2-AR, even though these agonists stimulate human cloned β_3-AR. A novel phenylethanolamine SB 215691 [(RS,RR)4-{2-[2-(3,4-dihydroxyphenyl)-2-hydroxyethylamino]propyl}phenoxymethyl)phosphonic acid mono(3-hydroxypropyl) ester] has now been identified, which has higher efficacy than BRL 37344 at human β_3-AR, and its lipolytic activity has been investigated.

Adenylyl cyclase activity ($n = 3$) was measured at 30°C in membranes from CHO cells that expressed 210, 559 and 390 fmol of human β_1, β_2- and β_3-AR (short form), respectively. Glycerol release ($n = 10$ patients) was measured at 37°C in human breast adipocytes (10–25 mg dry weight ml^{-1}). Phentolamine (10^{-6}M) was present in all the lipolysis experiments since SB 215691 appears to have α_2-AR agonist activity.

Table 1 EC_{50} values (nM) (intrinsic activities = IA)

	Cloned			Lipolysis
	β_1	β_2	β_3	
Isoprenaline	300 (1.0)	200 (1.0)	700 (1.0)	2.44 (1.0)
SB 215691	22 000 (0.48)	8300 (0.67)	520 (1.03)	100 (0.94)
BRL 37344	—(0.09)	9600 (0.34)	1300 (0.39)	
CGP 12177	—(0)	—(0)	400 (0.79)	126 (0.33)

The EC_{50} value for SB 215691 as a stimulant of lipolysis ranged from 12 to 380 nM and its pD_2 was positively correlated ($r = 0.94$, $P < 0.001$) with the IA of CGP 12177 (range 0.14–0.67) (Table 1). The pD_2 values of isoprenaline and CGP 12177 did not display this correlation ($P > 0.3$). In three experiments in which the IA of CGP 12177 was ≥ 0.44, nadolol (10^{-7} M) failed to shift the concentration–response curve for SB 215691, except at concentrations of SB 215691 that elicited a greater effect than the maximal response to CGP 12177. In other experiments, in which the CGP 12177 IA was ≤ 0.26, nadolol (10^{-7} M) did not shift the foot of the curve in a parallel fashion. In three experiments in the presence of 10^{-6} M nadolol the SB 215691 curve was biphasic, inflecting near the CGP 12177 maximal response. The apparent p$A_2 \pm$ SE for nadolol vs the isoprenaline response was 8.00 $\pm$ 0.03 ($n = 6$) for 10^{-7} M nadolol and 7.77 $\pm$ 0.21 ($n = 3$) for 10^{-6} M nadolol ($P < 0.05$).

These results indicate that a phenylethanolamine with high efficacy and selectivity for human cloned β_3-AR stimulates human adipocyte lipolysis via β_3-AR, its maximal effect via β_3-AR being similar to that of CGP 12177, and its potency being correlated with the β_3-AR responsiveness of the tissue. This is further evidence for functional β_3-AR in humans.

Index

Page numbers in bold indicate a main discussion; page numbers in italics indicate reference to an illustration or table.